WREN PUBLICATIONS

UNTWINNED: PERSPECTIVES (
THE DEATH OF A TWIN BEFOR.

ALTHEA HAYTON (EDITOR) is a graduate of Oxford
University and has worked at various times as a social
worker, adult education tutor and playgroup leader. She
has a diploma in counselling from the University of
Hertfordshire and has extensive experience of counselling
addicts and people with disabilities, including people with
cerebral palsy. She is founder and Project Director of
wombtwin.com, an informal non-profit-making organisation,
created to provide information, help and support to
wombtwin survivors around the world. She is sole proprietor
of Wren Publications and author of several non-fiction books,
notably *The Food Addicts Diet* (1991), *Not out of Mind*
(1998) and *Food and You* (2000). She is married with two
grown-up sons and lives in Hertfordshire, England.

# UNTWINNED: PERSPECTIVES ON THE DEATH OF A TWIN BEFORE BIRTH

**An anthology**

edited by

**Althea Hayton**

**Wren Publications**

Wren Publications
PO Box 396
St Albans
Herts
AL3 6NE
England

**ISBN 0-9525654-9-8**

Printed and bound in UK and USA by
Lightning Source

(UK office):
6 Precedent Drive, Rooksley
Milton Keynes Bucks, MK13 8PR

(US office):
1246 Heil Quaker Blvd.
la Verne TN 37086

# CONTENTS

# FOREWORD
## by
# DR LOUIS KEITH MD, PHD

*Dr. Louis G. Keith is an Emeritus Professor of Obstetrics
& Gynecology and recently retired as Professor of
Obstetrics and Gynaecology and Director of the Section of
Undergraduate Education and Medical Student Affairs at
Northwestern University Medical School in Chicago, having
worked there since 1975.*

*Because Dr. Keith is an identical (monozygotic) twin,
twinning has long been a major focus of his research
endeavours. He has spoken nationally and internationally
on a wide variety of subjects related to multiple pregnancy.
He is on the boards or advisory committees of numerous
international and United States organisations devoted to the
study of twins or the problems their families encounter.*

~~~~

Unlike the forewords to the other books I have written in the
past when I have known the author(s) for a number of years,
the author of this volume and myself have no connection,
other than the fact that we are both twins, she being a sole
survivor of a twin pregnancy and I being a co-survivor along
with my twin brother, Col. Donald M. Keith.

When I received the initial request to prepare a
foreword, along with the majority of the chapters, I was
intrigued to say the least, as I knew many of the authors
personally and had read their works over the years. I quickly
wrote a draft and left for a speaking engagement in the
Crimea where the other international speaker was Professor
Isaac Blickstein of Israel.

During one of his lectures, he put up a slide showing a pair of twins, one an-encephalic and the other normal, taken some hours before their birth by cesarean section. Professor Blickstein went on to note the tenderness in the facial expression of the an-encephalic co-twin, as if he were saying a final goodbye to his brother, knowing that they would be parted forever at the moment of their respective births and that he would not survive more than a few hours or days.

Looking at that picture, I recalled the famous picture, taken by David Teplica, MD, MFA, and which adorns the cover of our book *Iatrogenic Multiple Pregnancy,* of one-hour old twins where one is kissing the nose of the other. I further recalled that when I first saw it, it was apparent to me that this warm and loving behavior had to be a continuation of behavior that had been initiated in utero.

Similar thoughts were present on my part when I saw Professor Birgit Arabin's famous ultrasound, years ago at a meeting in Berlin, where the two twins were kissing lip to lip, on the one hand, or when one reached out and punched its so-twin. Simply stated, good reader, based on my personal observations (via ultrasound) of intrauterine behavior, I was well prepared to consider writing a foreword for this book, which explores yet another important facet of our knowledge base about twins, albeit one that the public may view with some degree of skepticism.

As readers well know, each book is unique, but this one is unique on several fronts. First and foremost, its content addresses an issue that is rarely, if ever, discussed in the scientific literature and for which there is little empirical or qualitative evidence. Second, it does so by melding together published works of a number of individuals in diverse fields who have written about the topic, albeit from totally different perspectives. To this are added the narrative experiences of survivors, again from differencing time frames of awareness and different degrees of acceptance. The "net result" has been the creation of "new information" that attempts to fill an obvious knowledge deficit.

Perhaps my viewpoint is biased, but even if this be the case, I do not feel that any apology is warranted. Not only am I an "identical" twin, but twinning has been part of my "professional activity" for decades, having attended countless meetings all over the world and having met countless sets of twins, some of whom were alone and recounted tales of a loss that they were reluctant to discuss with anyone who was themselves not a twin.

The overriding term to characterize Althea Hayton's newest work in this volume must be "scholarship" in its broadest context. Only someone devoted to the project and well read in all aspects of the now voluminous twin and multiple literature could have conceived it, let alone figured out what to include and what to ask for to be written, in order to fill in the gaps.

The book is divided into four parts. Part I "The Death of a Twin" contains seven chapters, many of them re-printed, which deal with a variety of points of view that describe and discuss the process of the death per se.

Part II, containing three re-printed chapters, deals with the "Vanishing Twin Phenomenon", not from the point of view that Professor Helain Landy and I have written about over the years (that is, that it is real, beyond the shadow of a doubt), but from other equally important viewpoints that reflect the effect of this phenomenon in the broader context of the world in which we live.

Part III (five chapters, some original and others re-printed) tackles the thorny topic of our ability to remember antenatal events. Although this has been described in the past, the amalgamation of five articles that deal with it in the context of twinship is unique.

The five original chapters of the book in Part IV are special because they deal with the heart of the problem, that is, the potential psychological effects on the survivor. Although placed at the end of the volume, they are a fitting beginning to new thoughts on this topic and further research in this area.

The publication of this book could not have come at a better time. The world is in the midst of an epidemic of Iatrogenic Multiple Pregnancies brought about mainly by the use of medical therapy that induces ovulation and the use of In Vitro Fertilization techniques. The majority of these pregnancies are di-tri-or quatri-zygotic, meaning that they arise from two, three or four fertilized eggs. The chance that one will die on its own or have to be reduced for the sake of the others is well known and accepted. Thus the potential number of "survivors" continues to grow year by year and the need for this book will expand in time.

The author is to be congratulated for her persistence in researching a difficult and little discussed topic which has broad social and ethical implications for all of society, considering that each set of twins, intact or with a death, is surrounded by two parents and two sets of grand parents to say the least. Society has been fascinated with twins since ancient times, and this volume goes to prove the veracity of Aristotle's comments that "Twins are outside nature's natural course - *Praeter Naturam*"

*Louis G. Keith, MD, PhD*
*Chicago, USA, 2006*

# INTRODUCTON

*Althea Hayton*

The effect on the survivor of losing a twin is largely underestimated, if not ignored. The focus, understandably enough, tends to be on the parents and their loss. Until about twenty years ago and the development of pre-natal psychology, it was generally assumed - if one thought about it at all - that there is no way a surviving twin would remember being with their twin in the first months of born life, let alone being in the womb with a co-twin who died early in pregnancy. It was thought that they would not miss or mourn for a twin they had never known.

The surviving twin has a very different inner experience of the loss, as can be seen in the early chapters of this book. It stretches the imagination somewhat to learn that a dead twin, who was presumably never known to the survivor, can be the subject of a sense of grief and loss, but clearly this is the case, at least for some. Furthermore, the way that society has chosen to ignore that loss only serves to add to this distress: until quite recently there has been no vocabulary, therapy or appropriate rituals of mourning for twin survivors.

To claim that one is a twin, when there is no physical proof that one's twin ever existed, is enough to disconcert anyone who relies solely on emprical data to establish the truth. To a scientist, attributing psychological problems such as depression, problems with food or suicidal thoughts to the loss of a twin many months before birth may seem at first glance to be misguided or even absurd. Yet I have chosen to make such a claim.

# INTRODUCTION

I have no physical proof that my twin ever existed, yet I believe I did indeed have a twin brother in the womb with me and he died about thirteen weeks into the pregnancy and was miscarried. I came to this realisation quite suddenly, with no proof except a deep, intuitive experience of the truth of this knowledge, which remains to me as real and sure as my own name.

I have in my long education been carefully schooled into applying scientific principles to any new idea. Therefore, I set out to prove this extraordinary idea scientifically, as far as I could. I quickly discovered "vanishing twin phenomenon" as I explored obstetrics, fetal development and embryogenesis. The more I tried to prove myself wrong, the more evidence appeared that I was probably right. At last I was convinced: I had a twin.

As a result of five years of research, I now have a list of indicators of a twin lost in pregnancy, which is growing ever longer as my research continues. Among these indicators are dermoid cysts, teratomas and genetic chimeras. There are unusual placentas, complicated pregnancies and premature birth. I have found fraternal twins, identical twins and mirror twins. I was told about additional fingers, ribs and bits of bowel - the residue of a lost twin. Then there is the *fetus in fetu* and the *fetus papyraceous*.

Proof that your twin was lost in the early weeks of life in the womb can of course only be found in the details of your mother's pregnancy. Sadly, many of these details are not recorded or not known. One must assume that this is because they were at the time considered to be of no medical interest or importance. Now that artifically assisted reproduction methods are being used so widely, every detail of these pregnancies is painstakingly noted. Every lost embryo, gradually fading away, is clearly visible on the ultrasound screen. This is incontrovertible proof.

For those without benefit of ultrasound, we have to look further for evidence of a missing twin. Clearly, there are many twin survivors who would be grateful for this medical evidence. It may simply be an announcement, usually made by mother, that they were once a twin. Parents and medical professionals are at last beginning to realise that this information is crucial to the psychological health of the survivor.

As I continue to explore, little snippets of seemingly unimportant evidence are beginning to cohere, and the possibility of a twin lost in the womb now seems quite reasonable. Even so, I know that for the survivor it is not the evidence that confirms the truth, but the inner understanding. I had no such evidence and no such announcement, yet one day I experienced that inner truth, alone in my own kitchen.

This single discovery has brought me here to day, working to articulate the vague and inchoate feelings and behaviours that seem to be characteristic of what I have called "wombtwin survivors" (i.e. the sole survivors of a twin or multiple pregnancy.) The central issue, as far as I am concerned, is not what may or may not have happened to me in the womb, but the persistent nature of my inner experience of a twin, created at a time when my brain and body were still being formed. It is not a memory exactly; it is too vague for that. It is more like a dream: a Dream of the Womb.

Four years ago I built the wombtwin.com website and began to work by email with two groups of visitors to the site. Firstly, there were those who knew about their twin already, but were just beginning to recognise that some of their psychological difficulties or problem behaviours might relate to this loss.

Secondly there was a smaller group, who stumbled on the wombtwin.com website because they had always had some vague intutive feeling that they may have had a twin, and needed someone to take them seriously. Some of these

3

people had been diagnosed as twin survivors by a therapist and needed some additional information, help and support.

This book arises directly out of this research. It is a collection of articles, some of which have been published elsewhere, but many of which have been written for me by a few of the people I have worked with.

We now have the words to make interpetations in terms of the Dream of the Womb. At last we can create a therapy that is useful for a surviving twin, whose twin was lost in in the first or second trimester of pregnancy. Some of the visitors to the website had been misdiagnosed as having a "personality disorder." It seems that some mental health professionals do not consider enquiring about a lost twin.

The therapy is simple: the idea of a twin lost in the womb is presented to the individual for consideration. If the twin is known, the loss is confirmed as a probable explanation for any difficult feelings, relationship problems or problem behaviours, such as overeating or self-abuse.

The next step is to provide the necessary information about life in the womb. It often happens that the survivor goes back to the family or seeks out medical or other evidence that their twin may have existed. If there is no such evidence, or if the individuals concerned are no longer available for comment, then the survivor must rely on their own intuitive sense of what happened.

Some survivors discover their twin in the process of psychotherapy or chiropractic treatment. Others seek confirmation through one of the new diagnostic therapies, One such is Neuro-Emotive Therapy, which appears to be particularly successful at finding vanished twins. Also, Family Constellation Therapy, created by Bert Hellinger and widely practiced for the benefit of families with relationship problems, often reveals a lost twin in the family, who has not been properly acknowledged or mourned. Once they have discovered and recognised their twin, many survivors find that simple fact to be enough : they need no other help. However, there are others who - for reasons that remain obscure at present - feel very needy and vulnerable. They need support and guidance through what I call the "wombtwin work," which is a kind of mentoring relationship. By means of this mentoring, the survivor can begin to understand the profound impact that this early loss has made upon their life. They grow stronger and become more autonomous.

For the participants in this process it feels like building an imaginary picture puzzle, but with no picture available as a guide. In the inner life of the survivor there are thousands of incidental and often very subtle behaviours, attitudes and beliefs that have seemed until now to be unrelated. As these coalesce around the idea of the missing twin, a vague picture begins to appear of *Someone Else There* who is also *Someone Gone Away.* The survivor becomes increasingly aware of how it felt to experience the loss of a twin and be left alone. The wombtwin work provides the vocabulary that enables the survivor to describe their feelings in a rational, logical way. It all makes perfect sense, and it is a great relief to know one is not crazy after all.

Knowing the exact nature of what happened in the womb is crucial to recovery, because that picture needs to be as clear as possible. For some, the idea of a lost twin is quite helpful but there seems to be a sticking point somewhere. In this case there may be more to discover and discuss before that all-important inner recognition is complete. So then we consider the possibility of other embryos present in those early months, or the traces of a previous miscarriage. There are so many variables and ramifications to consider about early life in the womb : we have a lot more to learn.

Two cases are described in this book that demonstrate the transformative nature of this work. In one case, nineteen years of anorexia ended in just six weeks. In another, a rational and logical reason was found for persistent suicidal thoughts in childhood.

Clearly, there is great healing potential in this idea and in this work. It seems that one in eight people is a surviving twin and at least a small proportion of these have a problem with this. We know that for some the loss of their twin is not much of a problem, but for others it will remain a major difficulty. A fear of abandonment, a painful sense of isolation and underlying depression are very common among surviving twins. That is quite reasonable when you consider that the survivor truly was abandoned, bereaved and left alone. Also common is low self esteem, addiction and suicidal thoughts. These too are predictable when we consider that the survivor has already known death in the womb - and may long to join their twin in death.

Collectively, these articles tell a story of a largely unacknowledged secret tragedy. However two books on the subject were published in Germany in 2006[1,2] so at last the idea is gaining ground. I hope that this volume will be the first of many, which will in time lay bare some of the physical and psychological difficulties associated with being a surviving twin.

## References:

1. Steinemann E. (March 2006) *Der verlorene Zwilling. Wie ein vorgeburtlicher Verlust unser Leben prägen kann.* (The vanished twin. How a prenatal loss can shape your life) Kösel-Verlag, München, Germany.

2. Austermann, A.R. ; Austermann, B. (May 2006) *Das Drama im Mutterleib. Der verlorene Zwilling,* (The drama in the womb. The vanished twin.) Königsweg, Berlin, Germany.

# PART ONE

## THE DEATH OF A TWIN
## AROUND BIRTH

# ANIM FORJINDAM

## REDISCOVERING MY TWIN

*My twin and I were born prematurely and my twin died shortly after birth. He was never spoken of. It was many years later that something deep in my spirit was awakened. At last I shed tears for my twin brother. I returned home to Cameroon and spoke to my mother, and my healing journey began.*

~~~~~

Anim Forjindam is a student of health sciences with a particular interest in pediatric surgery. She was born in Cameroon into a family with 8 sets of twins. Her twin brother died close to birth owing to a medical mistake.

*An original, previously unpublished article*
*© Anim Forjindam 2006*

# 1

## REDISCOVERING MY TWIN

*Anim Forjindam*

My name is Anim and my twin brother's name was Ngu. On October 20th 1983, my twin brother and I made our grand entrance into this world. We were born prematurely at a hospital in Cameroon. Shortly after birth, my brother was misdiagnosed and given a blood transfusion. This was a mistake that cost him his life and consequently rendered me twinless. Although the subject of twins evokes an enormous amount of interest and curiosity throughout our society, very little is known about twinless twins or womb twin survivors. Astonishingly, the infant mortality rate in twin pregnancies is six times higher than in regular pregnancies. Furthermore, in 20% of these births, one of the twins becomes a victim of Vanishing Twin Syndrome.

What happens when one twin dies and the other struggles to live? To what extent does this early loss shape the identity of the lone twin? Is it abnormal to spend hours crying for a twin that you have no tangible memories of? And when is it okay to shed the guilt of being a survivor and to embrace a new life of healing? Questions such as these plagued my mind for several years. This is the story of that bitter-sweet voyage towards letting go of the past, letting go of the pain, rediscovering my twin and ultimately finding happiness.

In West Africa, there are certain foods and traditional ceremonies reserved specially for twins. Growing up, my parents made sure that I partook of these twin customs. Ironically, my twin brother was hardly ever the subject of conversation. He was like the elephant in the room that everybody knows is there, but no one really talks about. I wanted to know why my family never put flowers on his tombstone on holidays or why he wasn't even mentioned on birthdays. However, at the risk of resurrecting old wounds, I buried my thoughts and remained silent.

Eventually, I moved away from home to the United States to get a better education. As an honor student, I went through high school like any normal teenager just trying to fit in. When my friends would ask me what my name meant, instead of telling them that 'Anim' was an African twin name, I told them that it was just a regular name, void of any special meaning. In reality, I think I was simply too ashamed to admit that I was twinless. After my senior year, I went off to college to be an engineer. I eventually discovered my passion for medicine and made up my mind to become a doctor. In between being the president of the American Pre-Medical Student Association , secretary of the African student association, a singer in a Christian gospel group and doing volunteer work in the community, I some how managed to excel in all my classes that semester.

My juggling act at school would soon come tumbling down. The breaking point occurred at a weekend retreat while serving as a grief counselor to children coping with the death of a loved one. The event began with a candle lighting ceremony and at that moment, something deep in my spirit was awakened. A something that I can only describe as an aching heart. For the first time in my life, I shed tears for my twin brother. A Pandora's Box of emotions that I could neither shut nor walk away from had been unlocked. I was angry at myself for being the twin who had lived. I was upset with my family for moving on and acting as if he had never existed. I was bitter at Ngu for abandoning me when I needed him the most.

I was even angry at God for allowing him to die. Why did it have to be my twin brother and why was I the only one crying for Ngu?

I refrained from verbalizing my feelings to anyone because I honestly didn't understand how it was possible to be so distraught over someone I barely even knew. Nothing seemed to make sense anymore and there were days when I wondered if I was losing my mind. As time went on, my mind became increasingly troubled and I found it impossible to concentrate on my school work. In the fall of my junior year in college, I did something that was very hard for me. I obtained permission from the school and I withdrew for the year. I had decided to go home to my family in Cameroon. Perhaps returning to the motherland, where lay Ngu's bones, would end this bizarre behavior and give me the closure that I so desperately desired.

The journey back to my country was therapeutic. I finally got the opportunity to talk to my family about Ngu. To my greatest surprise, I discovered that my mother and I shared something very striking in common. We were both surviving twins. Unfortunately, my mother's twin sibling was miscarried during the second trimester of the pregnancy. With this new knowledge, I was able to open up and relate to my mother on a more intimate level. In a strange way, our past tragedies had brought us closer together than we could have ever imagined. All the anger and hurt in my heart was soon replaced with forgiveness and gratitude.

As I returned to the United States to resume my studies, I felt as though a huge load had been lifted off my shoulders. Despite the fact that I was ready to get back to my old enthusiastic self, there was just one little problem: I still felt trapped in a bottomless pit of despair. Although I knew that I had to let go of all my emotional baggage and say goodbye to Ngu, what I didn't know, was how to love the person staring back at me in the mirror.

11

I continued to inflict upon myself, the pressure of "living for two" in order to make up for my twin's death. In addition, I set impossibly high goals to camouflage the guilt that festered inside of me. Perhaps I had cheated my twin brother of life and like the Greek mythology figure Sisyphus, I was doomed to carry this burden on my shoulders for all eternity. As an African woman, my parents had raised me to be courageous and independent. How could I possibly tell them that I had contracted the "blue pill disease" known as depression? For anyone who has ever been on the brink of despair, there comes a *kairos* moment when you realize that if you don't do something NOW, tomorrow will be too late. I knew that I couldn't do this on my own, so I sought professional help from a bereavement counselor.

As she was an expert in the field of psychology and research pertaining to twin loss, I began an eye opening correspondence with the counselor. I came to understand that a lot of the character traits and emotions that I was experiencing at the time were common amongst twin survivors. Due to the fact that my own twin had never been fully acknowledged, I was manifesting the symptoms of "blocked grief" and essentially going through a delayed mourning process. Based on her own twin research, she had discovered that twin survivors tend to be very empathetic, intuitive and creative. While they are often charming and work hard to keep others happy, twin survivors also posses some destructive behavior patterns. They start many things at once but seldom finish. They are over achievers who tend to always be busy and in search of new ideas. They are looking for something or someone that can never be found. They are looking for their missing twin. It dawned on me that I was not alone in my search for answers.

More importantly, my counselor helped me realize that I was not crazy after all. After all these years of questioning my identity, I have finally learned to stop crying for my twin and start celebrating who I am. My twin brother's death may have been an accident but my life doesn't have to be one as well. Instead of seeing myself as a twin-LESS twin, I have chosen to see myself through the loving eyes of The One who created me: Strong not Weak, Victorious not a Victim, Free not Fearful, Proud of who I am today and who I'll be tomorrow. Not Ashamed of the past. I used to think that I was justified in being angry and bitter; after all hadn't I been robbed of my birthright as a twin? I know now, that as long as I continue to focus on what I have lost, I will never overcome the problem. However, if I dare to look beyond my circumstances and grasp hold of how much I already posses, I will find my solution. I will find a happiness that is not limited by obstacles and only then, will I begin to tap into the incredible reservoir of courage and strength that lives inside of me.

These days when people ask me what my name means, I proudly tell them that Anim is a Cameroonian twin name. I am going to school full time to pursue my dream of becoming a pediatric surgeon and I am also training for my very first marathon. As I run my race, the important thing isn't receiving first place or breaking a record. My satisfaction comes from simply crossing that finish line and doing the best that I can. There are millions of surviving twins in the world who are still hurting. If after reading my story, I am able to help even one person let go of the pain and find their own unique path towards healing, then these words would have served their purpose.

# ELIZABETH A. PECTOR  MD

## TWIN TRADITIONS WORLDWIDE FOR LIFE, DEATH AND MOURNING

*The grief journey for a bereaved twin varies greatly throughout the world. However, universal themes include the uniqueness and vulnerability of multiples, the enduring status of twinship, and a close relationship that requires balance and special attention to a lone twin's needs. The examples presented here may help lone twins develop their own traditions to honor their irreplaceable companions.*

~~~~~

Dr. Pector is a board certified family physician practising in the Naperville area since 1987.  Dr. Pector has researched many aspects of multiple birth and prematurity and published and spoken on related topics.  The death of one of Dr. Pector's twin sons inspired much of her research and her continued interest in multiple-birth issues.

*Adapted from: Twin death and mourning worldwide: a review of the literature. Twin Research 2002;5(3):196-205.*

# 2

## TWIN TRADITIONS WORLDWIDE FOR LIFE, DEATH AND MOURNING

*Elizabeth A. Pector*

For thousands of years, twins and higher multiples have attracted curiosity and awe. They inspired colorful myths among natives of Europe, the Americas, Asia and Africa. Based on such legends, fascinating traditions emerged. Some twin customs faded away long ago, but many remain part of modern life.

When one or both twins died, many funerary rituals honored the twins' unique nature and their special relationship with their co-twins, their earthly clan and the spirit world. The survey of twin traditions presented here may inspire modern lone twins to creatively memorialize their wombmates.

### A multitude of beliefs

Around the world, cultural opinions of twins and multiples have ranged from godly to evil, and sometimes both views have existed within a single culture. Regardless of prevailing attitudes, societies have often recognized multiples as special, rare, and fragile, requiring elaborate, careful treatment.

Some cultures believed multiples have close connections to the gods. The Mohave Indians in North America and several western and southern African tribes considered twins to be heavenly visitors. Twin paternity was attributed to a mountain or sea god by Giljak and Ainu peoples on Sakhalin Island in far eastern Russia.

Human multiples were sometimes felt to have a kinship with animals that bear litters of two or more offspring. Twins have been linked to birds, bears, bushcows, salmon, snakes, lizards, and monkeys. Moreover, many cultures have believed that multiples have magical effects on the fertility of crops, animals and humans; power over thunder, lightning and rain; or ability to change into animal form. Some peoples feared the spirits of deceased multiples could adversely affect the luck of their families and community, so they carefully appeased twin spirits during special celebrations.

Regrettably, evil origins were sometimes attributed to multiples, with cultures asserting that one or both twins were conceived through the mother's infidelity with another man or a spirit, animal, or devil. Sinful relations were attributed to boy-girl twins in some civilizations, where the babies were thought to have violated a prohibition against incest—while still in the womb! Some societies considered multiples and their parents to be taboo and forced them to live apart from the main settlement and to atone for a multiple birth, even if one or more of the babies died.

Vanished or hidden twins have been important in both Africa and the West. For instance, the southeast African Karanga believed bleeding near the time an expectant mother's missed menstrual period, called *kukamura* - "to divide or halve"- meant an unwanted twin had been aborted by ancestors. In western Africa, Kedjom culture attributes misfortunes to hidden twinship, and prescribes expensive rituals to escape misused twin powers. As this region has grown more distressed economically, shamans discern a rising number of occult twins. In the West, vanishing twins are invoked to explain loneliness in what Hillel Schwartz calls a "culture of the copy," where modern man is surrounded by duplications, imitations and virtual realities. Amidst these frequent facsimiles, Schwartz suggests that

we may seek in a vanished twin both an assurance of
faithfulness and an eternal human connection.  At the same
time, vanished twinship may also serve as a vehicle for
feelings of inexpressible loss. [1]

## Precautions to promote twin survival

Many societies took pains to prevent the sorrowful loss of
their special twin children.  Developing countries, as well
as industrialized nations, have long known that twins are at
risk of arriving small and weak, with higher mortality rates
than singletons.  Such views were expressed in places as
widely  separated as Alaska, Ecuador, Africa, the Himalayas,
Malaysia and Indonesia.  The Toradja of Indonesia went
so far as to separate boy-girl twins at birth to prevent one
from stealing the other's life spirit.  Among many cultures,
one child was expected to die soon after the other if proper
traditions were not observed after the first child's death.

To prevent their new arrivals from quickly departing,
societies have used a number of strategies.   The first is
preferential treatment for multiples.  Among the Yorubans
in western Africa, who have a highly developed cult that
regards twins as embodied deities, fathers of newborn twins
will respectfully prostrate themselves before their infants so
they will not "go back."  Similarly, the west African Dogon
and Kpe, and Native American Chippewa, Mohave, and
Yuma tribes feared that twins might return to their heavenly
home if they did not like the home or family, if they were
disciplined, if they were not promptly picked up, or if they
envied another child conceived before weaning the twins.
To counteract such capricious behavior, the Oku of
Cameroon observe a birth ritual for twins, and believe they
will only thrive if they are given brown salt and palm oil.
Meanwhile, the Bambara and Malinke elsewhere in West
Africa offer twins meat, eggs and milk that would ordinarily
be reserved for adult men.  Similarly, Yoruban feasts for

17

twins involve special foods: palm oil, kola nuts, ground maize, bananas, and fowl, plus beans to calm the twins' temper. Parents of Igbo and Yoruban twins in Nigeria, like the Yokuts in America, received monetary gifts from others to keep the twins strong. Yoruban mothers often dance and sing about their twins in the marketplace and receive money from onlookers.

As a second precaution, twins have sometimes been kept away from strangers or mourners. Navajo parents protected twins from strangers, and southwest African Mbundu mothers of triplets shook rattles at passers-by to keep their babies from dying. The Dogon kept mourners from entering a twin birth hut, and fathers of twins would not attend funerals. South African Thonga twin children were considered frail, but were allowed to visit a mourning family if their heads were first smeared with ashes by the gravedigger.

A third strategy to protect multiple-birth children is religious and medicinal customs. The Rundi in central Africa performed ceremonies to prevent twins from dying. Kedjom mothers in western Africa administer medicines throughout twins' lives to strengthen them. Yoruban parents consult a diviner to learn the desires of their twins for foods, sacrifices, rituals and taboos that will ensure their survival. Haitians held festivals every few years, *mange marassa*, to honor both living and dead multiples. Living twins wore costly, identical new clothes, and food was offered to deceased multiples' spirits in double and triple bowls to prevent misfortune. In French Guiana (South America), special twin dances were held every 4 to 5 years to avoid angering the spirits of deceased twins.

A fourth, and common, strategy for ensuring the survival of multiples is scrupulously equal treatment of all the children. The Bukidnon of the Phillipines observed a ritual exchange of rings between the babies at birth, to maintain a balance between them. Several tribes in North American and Africa believed that multiples needed identical treatment to avert fatal jealousy. The Toradja in Indonesia never disciplined identical twins, afraid that both would fall ill. Conversely, the Nkundu in central Africa punished all the multiples, even if only one deserved it. The Nkundu took great care to give even the smallest objects identically to each child and to carry both at the same time. Likewise, the Mohave in North America would give twins identical presents. The Sinkaietsk in Northwest North America dressed multiples alike. The Nootka from the same region took the additional precaution of nursing both twins at the same time and put them down to rest in identical cradles, but facing away from each other so they could not talk together and conspire to go back to "Salmon's Home." One Hawsa-speaking Mawri woman in west Africa felt that merely discussing size differences between twins would prompt the smaller to kill the larger.

Identical treatment during adolescence among the African Bomvana extended so far as mock circumcision for a boy's twin sister! She shaved her head like her brother, exchanged a necklace with him, and sat beside him. The operator pretended to circumcise her first before moving on to her brother. While the boy was secluded in the circumcision hut, she wore one of his shirts. Likewise, Tallensi twins in Ghana in western Africa were considered equal, "one yet two." A pair of male twins among the Tallensi would live together for life; two Tallensi sisters would marry within a same or adjacent settlement. When one of a female set of twins married among either the AmaXosa or Bomvana, both young women donned matching wedding dresses to puzzle the groom. When the second sister married, the first returned to repeat the charade. Among the Nuer, when the firstborn of a male twin pair married, both brothers entered the groom's hut to strike the bride on the head before the younger brother exited.

## Funerary rituals

*Twin souls: Two, or one?*
In many places around the world--Europe, Asia, Africa,
Indonesia, North America—twins were believed to share
a single soul, to be of "one breath," halves of a whole,
one spirit in two bodies. Two Native American tribes, the
Tlingit and Yuma, felt the twin bond and risk of death for a
surviving twin was only important in childhood. The Tlingit
asserted that twins "breathed for each other" until about
10 years of age. Birth order was important to Eskimos,
who felt that a firstborn twin's death foretold the younger
twin's demise, but that the eldest could survive death of the
second-born. The Jicarilla in New Mexico believed twins
were two people sharing one life. Thus, if one died, the
other's life would also be shortened. Similarly, the Karanga
in southeast Africa asserted that a surviving twin would
die of loneliness. Competition or revenge appears in other
traditions. The Mohave in America believed that twins were
immortal visitors from heaven, and that boy-girl twins had
been married to each other in heaven. It was feared that if
opposite-sex twins quarreled, one might die, followed soon
thereafter by the offended "spouse." Similarly, the Chippewa
believed that a mistreated twin who died would soon be
followed by the equally dissatisfied wombmate.

Given the pervasive beliefs about the risk of a
surviving twin's death, when one twin died, precautions
were sometimes taken to prevent the survivor's soul from
following his or her wombmate into the afterlife. The
Yorubans administered medications to the living child to
prevent him or her from seeing or hearing the twin who died.
The Sumba in Indonesia ritually separated the soul to avoid
death of the surviving child. Likewise, among the Karen
people in former Burma, a lone twin's wrist would be bound

with a cord to prevent the soul from escaping. The Mossi
in western Africa considered infant twins to be malicious,
less-than-human bush spirits until a subsequent sibling was
born. However, if one twin died, the survivor was ritually
"pegged" or fastened to life and thereafter regarded as fully
human. Residents of Galoa Island in Fiji considered the
survivor to be dead until complex ceremonies revived him.

Among some peoples, death was only mentioned
euphemistically so as not to harm the living twin. The
AmaXosa in south Africa would say that a deceased twin
was pretending, married, torn from his fellow, or broken off.
The Yorubans in Nigeria, with a well-developed twin cult,
would say that a twin who passed away had "gone to Lagos"
(the Nigerian capital) to bring his parents wealth. The Nuer
in eastern Africa, who feel that twins are kin to birds, explain
that dead twins have "flown away." This expression is also
used by the Dogon in western Africa and Baganda in central
Africa.

Similarly, some cultures felt it was inappropriate to
mourn for a twin who died. This was true among Zulus in
southern Africa, who did not favor twins. They believed that
expressing sorrow for a twin would anger the community
ancestral spirit. A Native American woman did not want
the deceased child's name spoken so his spirit would not be
called back from its peaceful resting place. The Nootka of
northwestern North America considered it taboo to sorrow at
a twin's passing.

Nuer twins also did not mourn if one twin died, because
they believed they shared a single soul and personality. An
adult Nuer woman whose twin had died pointed out, "Is not
his soul still living? I am alive, and we are really children of
God."[2]

*Special ceremonies*
When funeral rites were observed, they often reflected the

unique nature attributed to twins. For instance, when a
South African AmaXosa twin died, he exchanged a blanket,
beads and clothes with the deceased, who was buried in the
survivor's clothes. Prior to his twin's burial, the survivor lay
briefly in the grave while wearing the dead twin's clothing.
Family members did not shave their heads or mourn until
the surviving twin passed away. The AmaXosa did not
work in their fields for two days after a twin's death due
to the community's sorrow. Loss of both twins was tragic,
and anyone who hoed too soon afterward could expect a
hailstorm to destroy their crops!

Some twins were accorded great respect when they died.
The Bangolan in west African Cameroon bury twins like a
king on a throne. The Azande buried them at a roadside,
where travelers could toss grass, a leaf or stick on the grave
to bring good luck. The Wanyoro in east Africa observed
a long mourning period after death of a twin, and gave
deceased twins their own miniature huts. The Giljak on
Sakhalin Island ordinarily cremated singletons, but twins and
their parents were buried. Twins, thought to be children of
the mountain god, were dressed in white and seated Turkish
style in a specially built house.

Some twin-animal associations influence funeral rituals.
The Ga in west Africa believed that twins have the wild
bushcow's spirit, thus living twins ran around like wild cows
after a twin died. Since the Nootka felt that twins had close
affinity to salmon, they were not buried but were laid on
swampy ground. Older Nootka twins were placed in a box
in a riverside tree until the current ultimately swept away
box and tree together. The Nuer in Africa felt that twins, like
birds, are children of gods who dwell in clouds. A stillborn
twin was placed in a basket in a tree, with the assumption
that birds of prey would know they were kin and leave the
body intact.

Supposed twin powers over weather affected rites in two cultures. The Thonga in south Africa felt a twin birth was a disaster that threatened drought. To counteract this, deceased twins would be buried in wet ground. During a drought, previously buried twins might be exhumed and reburied at lower elevation. Among the Aymara of Bolivia, one poor family in the 1960s could not afford an elaborate twin burial ritual. When it hailed the following week, leaders were summoned from neighboring towns to conduct a service that mingled Catholic and native traditions to prevent curses, grief and disgrace and bring health to the twins' souls.

The special status of twins endures after they pass away. After death of both infant twins, a more somber Ugandan Baganda twin naming feast was still held without the usual dancing, singing and drumming. Mbuti pygmy mothers of twins, in central Africa, still carried out their traditional dances if their twins died at birth. If one Cameroon Oku twin dies, the survivor still receives the special twin rite. When one of Dogon twins died, the survivor's first birthday feast was celebrated at the first birthday of the subsequent child, who was named for the deceased twin. The Ga in Ghana, Yorubans, Haitians and others continued twin rituals after their death. An iron fetish called a *sinzin* was hung in the home of Bambara twin parents to house the genie of twins. Annual sacrifices were made to it long after twins had both died.

## Tangible mementos: effigies bring comfort

Special objects have been used to memorialize deceased twins in places as diverse as North America, Sakhalin Island, and throughout Africa. Such objects include bracelets, gourds, and most notably, human figurines. In Africa, these have included carved statuettes, sticks or store-bought dolls. The Papago in North America carved two figures after one twin's death. One figure was buried with the deceased, the other kept with the survivor to prevent loneliness. Similarly, in the African Congo and among southeast African Ovimbundu, effigy figures were buried with surviving twins when they died.

The Giljak near Japan carved one figure (two figures joined at the sides if both died) and placed them in a model *yurt* (hut). Daily food offerings were carried out for three generations, until the figures were brought atop a mountain for a final sacrificial offering. A stick three to six feet long, carved with a curly design, was planted in the ground next to the model *yurt* to save the community from haunting by the twins' spirits. At the time of a lone twin's marriage, the African Bambara and Malinke carved another figure to represent the deceased twin's spouse. Both statues were kept together in the married couple's home.

Yorubans have become particularly famous for their skillful *ibeji* carvings that serve as a home for a deceased twin's half-soul. The bereaved parents consult a diviner, who selects a carver to fashion a statuette. These carvings include tribal facial marks but are not realistic portraits. Shoulders appear strong, arms are long, and prominent breasts or male genitalia suggest an adult spirit in the prime of life. The heads are colored with indigo dye, and the bodies are often rubbed with camwood powder, which is also commonly used to prevent illness in small children. Cowry shells or strands of beads around the neck, waist, wrist or ankles of the figure are added for adornment. *Ibeji* figurines are treated the same as any surviving multiples throughout life, carried by the mother throughout her daily routines, put to breast at the same time as the living child, "fed" bits of food, laid to rest at night beside the survivor, and frequently rubbed with special oils. Weekly rituals begin with calling out the name of the deceased, singing, and presenting food such as bean cakes and palm oil to the figure. Annual celebrations include dances at which mothers of twins will wrap the *ibeji* figures in their belts or grasped tightly in their hands. When the surviving twin comes of age, he or she cares for the statue and observes the proper rituals.

## Final thoughts

The grief journey for a bereaved twin varies greatly throughout the world. However, universal themes include the uniqueness and vulnerability of multiples, the enduring status of twinship, and a close relationship that requires balance and special attention to a lone twin's needs. The examples presented here may help lone twins develop their own traditions to honor their irreplaceable companions.

~~~~~

## References

1. Schwartz H. (1998)*The culture of the copy: striking likenesses, unreasonable facsimiles*. Zone Books: New York. p.21

2. Evans-Pritchard EE. (1936) Customs and beliefs relating to twins among the Nilotic Nuer. *Uganda Journal* 3:230-8.

## Further reading

Belo J. A study of customs pertaining to twins in Bali. (1935) *Tijdschrift voor Indische Tall-Land-en Volkenkunde* 75:484-549.

Chemeche G.(2003) *Ibeji: the cult of Yoruba twins*. 5 Continents Editions, Milan

Devereux G. Mohave (1941) beliefs concerning twins. *American Anthropologist (News Series)* 43, 473-542.

Diduk S. (1993) Twins, ancestors and socio-economic change in Kedjom society. *Man (New Series)* 28(3):551-71.

Imperato PJ. (1971) Twins among the Bambara and Malinke of Mali. *Journal of Tropical Medicine and Hygiene* 74(7), 154-9.

Leroy F. (1976) Attitudes toward twinning in primitive societies. *Acta Geneticae Medicae et Gemellologicae* 25:20-3.

Leroy F, (2002) Olaleye-Oruene T, Koeppen-Schomerus G, Bryan E. Yoruba customs and beliefs pertaining to twins. *Twin Research* 5(2): 132-6.

*Parabola Magazine* (1994) Twins: the two who come from one. 19(2).

Pector EA. (2002) Twin death and mourning worldwide: a review of the literature. *Twin Research* 5(3):196-205.

Renne EP, Bastian ML.(2001) Reviewing twinship in Africa. *Ethnology* 40(1):1-11.

~~~~~

# FOOTPRINTS

Tiny feet
That should be taking baby steps
Instead left
Giant Footprints
Embedded in my heart.

Matching Feet
Now walking, take their baby steps
Alone.

They should have walked together
But only one will blaze a trail
His trailhead marked by
Giant Footprints
Left there by his stillborn twin:
Buried wombmate memories that linger deep within.

*Elizabeth Pector*

~~~~~

*Jared Scott and Bryan Samuel Pector, identical twin boys,
were born by urgent Cesarean at 33 weeks gestation in
February, 1997, five hours after Bryan was
found dead on a "routine" ultrasound.*

*Footprints was written in fall 1998,
when Jared was learning to walk.*

# AUDREY SANDBANK

## …AND THEN THERE WAS ONE

*The loss of a child at any age brings heartbreak as there are
so many might-have-beens but the loss of a twin is somehow
perpetuated in the survivor. Bereaved parents need to feel
their grief is acknowledged, and the surviving twin needs
to know that he or she is not responsible. The whole
family needs to understand that the lost co-twin is an
ever present reality.*

~~~~~

Audrey Sandbank is married with a son and twin daughters.
She is a UKCP registered family psychotherapist and
has practiced family therapy for twenty years as part of a
multi-disciplinary team. Audrey is now in private practice
in Surrey. For the last fifteen years she has been Hon.
Consultant Family Therapist to the Twins and Multiple
Births Association. She is author of *Twins and the Family*,
a parenting manual, based on her own research and clinical
practice, and editor of *Twin and Triplet Psychology – A
professional guide to working with multiples*. She helped
to set up the "Young Minds" Parents Information Service
Helpline and is currently one of the professional advisors
providing a professional ringback service. She is a regular
writer and broadcaster.

*Extract from book: Twins and the Family (Chapter 16)
Published by TAMBA (Twins and Multiple Births Association)
Revised edition, 2003*

# 3

## ...AND THEN THERE WAS ONE

*Audrey Sandbank*

### The bereaved parents

The loss of a child at any stage brings heartbreak as there
are so many might-have-beens, but the loss of a twin is
somehow perpetuated in the survivor. There is also the loss
of something that is not given to everyone: the privilege of
having two babies, an achievement that is out of the ordinary.

The way that hospital staff react to the death of a
stillborn or newborn twin is of great importance. The birth
of twins in the maternity ward is always exciting and staff
may deal with their own feelings of loss by denying those
of the parents. They may also feel that parents should be
grateful that they have one healthy baby when others, less
fortunate, have none. The mother and father may be given
the message that it is unacceptable to grieve. The baby is
unceremoniously disposed of as though it had never existed.

The grief may come later and be diagnosed as post-natal
depression, or be delayed until the birth of the next baby.
All parents need to know and understand about the death of
their baby. If a stillborn baby is damaged in some way, the
parents' imagination may be far worse than the reality. If
they can see and hold the dead baby and talk to someone
who is in a position to answer their questions, they will find
it easier to come to terms with the death.

Dr Elizabeth Bryan[1] has found that a photograph of
a baby that is stillborn or who dies before it can be taken
home can be of tremendous solace to parents and later to a

surviving twin. It will also help to separate the two babies in the mother's mind. Even a picture of the final scan can be helpful. Parents need to know whether their babies were identical or non-identical. If parents are able to nurse their sick baby in hospital, even if it only has a brief time to live, a great deal of loving and caring can be given during its short life and parents can feel they did all they could for their baby. This can make it easier to let him go, and if there is a surviving twin the parents can be freed to love the remaining baby. However, before they can do so the parents need some space to grieve on their own. Perhaps the mother could be moved to a smaller side ward and given extra visiting time to be with her husband and family. The importance of parents sharing their grief cannot be emphasized too much, or each may build a wall around their feelings which can cause lasting damage to their relationship. If there is no period of mourning, the grief may return later under a different guise.

Hospitals can sometimes be in too much of a hurry to dispose of a dead baby and, in the midst of their grief, many parents do not realize that they could have a small ceremony and a proper burial. Parents have said that they have sometimes doubted the reality of the second baby, but a shared service and a tiny grave, or perhaps a rose bush planted in the garden of remembrance can give their memory a focal point.

After the first shock and disbelief, feelings of anger may be uppermost in the parents' minds. Why did the doctors not save him? Why did they not respond to signals from the mother that something was wrong? Endless questions that need patient answers. Sometimes the parents' anger may be turned against the partner or against the surviving twin. What right had he to survive when his twin died? He must have been too greedy, to big, a cuckoo in the nest destroying his brother. The dead twin becomes idealized, perfect, deserving of love, the survivor undeserving, a usurper, the bad baby. If a mother becomes stuck in her anger then professional help will usually assist her to move on, but the anger is a natural stage in grieving and, if understood and shared, will gradually decrease. A mother who is aware of her feelings towards the surviving baby, but finds them unacceptable, may compensate by over-indulging the child so that he becomes powerful and difficult. She is unable to be firm but finds it progressively harder to control her angry feelings. He becomes the bad child of her imagination.

Once the mother understands that these feelings are normal and will pass and that she is not helping the surviving child by indulging him, she can begin to set limits and refuse to respond to bids for negative attention. Good behaviour is rewarded with praise. Once the child has learned that 'no' means 'no' and has found how he can please his mother, a loving relationship can grow and the child will be freed from a growing belief in his own badness.

Another aspect of grief is loss of faith in life itself, a loss of confidence that a child can survive or that the parent is able to protect him. This loss of confidence can be seen in children who have lost one parent and who will not let the other parent out of their sight. This same instinct may cause a parent to over-protect the surviving child, particularly after a cot death of one twin. It is known that there is a greater risk to the surviving twin, but this is principally within the first few days, and parents can feel more confident once a month has passed. However, even when the co-twin died at birth and the survivor is a healthy baby, parents may transmit their worries and fears to him.

Surviving twins are sometimes said to be lonely children, but a child who lacks confidence in himself will often find it difficult to make friends. He may also be child who finds it hard to cope with the rough and tumble of the playground.

Loving parents can find it difficult to be cross or deny the child what he wants if he is a precious survivor, and this, too, can contribute to difficulties that he may have in making relationships.

For a child to feel really secure, he needs limits and guidelines and parents who have faith that he will be able to deal with life. Even if they feel that he is vulnerable, they can sometimes manage to disguise their feelings and give him a little push into the world. If he feels that his parents believe in him he will surprise them and himself and all concerned will gain a real sense of confidence in his ability to tackle life on his own.

Sudden death always carries a stronger sense of guilt, whoever it is, at whatever age. The endless self-questioning. Even more so in the case of a cot death, where there simply are no answers to be found, and yet they are continually sought. The parents feel that if they can find answers then perhaps they can protect the other twin; without answers, who can help him? And there is the guilt of things left undone that could have been done, of having been tired and perhaps irritable and impatient with a child irretrievably lost. Of not having picked up the cuddly toy the day before when he dropped it.

If we are given a little time to show we care and make our peace it is easier to live with ourselves afterwards. This is why it is so important for parents to have the opportunity of nursing a dying child or baby. It is important, too, for the other children in the family to make their farewells.

It can be helpful to have a loving mother figure in the house, such as a grandmother or a sister, to enable the parents to have time to grieve whilst young children and the co-twin baby can continue to feel good and lovable.

'Michael only came to visit, he couldn't stay, but John will stay and be your baby brother,' might be a helpful explanation for a three-year-old who could feel that his bad feelings had hurt the baby, or that he had somehow wished him away.

When twins are identical, parents sometimes feel that by offering the survivor the love that they would have given to his twin - in other words, by giving him twice the love - they are in some way giving what they owe to the dead baby. They are also acknowledging the survivor's loss. There can often be a special relationship between these survivors and their parents. It is possible that even such young children feel some of the guilt of the survivor – 'Why me?' - and try to justify their survival through their own lives.

The identical twin is more than a reminder of the dead twin. The parents know how the baby would have looked, or even behaved, if he had lived. The lost non-identical town is remembered at every birthday, but would he perhaps have been more successful, more loving, not have spoken to his parents like that? If one of a boy/girl pair, might he have been more of a companion, someone to share things with, the son, or daughter they never had? The surviving twin may live constantly under the shadow of the dead one, feeling that he can never be good enough.

Parents who have lost a single baby can sometimes find solace, if they have been allowed sufficient space to grieve for the first, in the birth of their next baby. This baby can never replace the first, but it can help to heal the wound if the decision to have another child has not been taken too quickly and the child is wanted for himself.

For parents of twins this is impossible. A new baby can never restore his companion to the surviving twin or the dream of being the proud parents of twins. There is also the loss for the parents and the surviving twin of that precious

enjoyment of each other in the first few months of life,
perhaps longer, because of the shadow of the lost baby.

There are now many self-help groups for parents who
have lost a baby, and the local Twins Club will put parents
who have lost a twin in touch with others who have
experienced a similar loss. Although going to meetings and
seeing parents who have both their twins may be too painful.
Talking and sharing with others can be the greatest help in
the long term. If the baby dies at birth or soon after, then
the talking begins in the hospital, sharing memories with
the hospital staff and then continuing at home with family
and friends. If it is a cot death, then the doctor and health
visitor may be an added source of comfort and reassurance.
But parents who have suffered a similar loss may be the ones
who have the most to offer.

## The lone twin

There is reason to believe that if a twin is lost during
pregnancy, the survivor may be aware of his loss, even
if only at an unconscious level, and may feel some
responsibility.

If the lost twin is sometimes talked about it will not only
help the parents, but help the child. The child's feelings and
fears can be expressed and parents may be able to reassure
him. The example of the seedlings which do not all grow in
the window box or garden can be shown not be the fault of
the ones that do, but one of the happenings of nature.

The longer the twins both survive, the greater the shock
to the survivor when his co twin dies. Young twins may
show the same separation anxiety when a co-twin has to go
into hospital, as a child will show when separated from his
mother. The shock of a cot death will affect all the family,
but it can affect a twin's basic trust in the world around him.
If the parents are overcome with grief then there may be a

need for a temporary mother figure, but many parents find that the needs of the survivor help them through this difficult time.

Because a young baby has difficulty distinguishing himself from the world about him, the 'me' from the 'not me', he may believe that others have the same feelings as himself: 'If I love, I am loved, if I hate, I am hated.' If he then has angry feelings towards the twin with whom he is sharing his mother and the twin dies, he may not only have feelings of guilt but feelings that he may be punished.

Photographs of both twins together (for the twin that is bereaved at birth, taken in the hospital if possible) will help the survivor to see his twin as someone separate from himself, and if later the death is talked about and he learns to understand that he was in no way responsible, he will be helped to come to terms with the death.

The belief of a child that he has magical abilities is greatest between the ages of three and five, and a twin who is unfortunate enough to lose his partner at this time may feel deeply responsible and invite punishment.

The greatest help that can be given to a child of this age is to give a great deal of love, without letting the child take the control from the parents, and to give no negative attention. In this way the child learns that he is 'good' and that he is not able to be destructive. The temptation can be to give in to a bereaved toddler in order to make up to him for his loss, but this will increase his sense of omnipotence. If parents are finding difficulty in handling the child, they may be advised to seek help from the child and adolescent services.

Talking and sharing is important too, although it may be painful to the parents. The child's questions can then be answered and his fears brought out into the open. Long adult discussions should be avoided. However, in the case of twins, language may not yet be sufficiently developed for much discussion to take place at the time and talking may come later.

The closer the twin pair, the greater the distress when one twin dies, at whatever age. For the identical twin, there may be a shock that is similar to losing a limb. If twins have been helped to find a sense of personal identity during childhood, with their own individual friends and interests as well as those in common, they will have some support to help them with the trauma of what may seen like the loss of half of themselves. Nothing can lessen their grief, but it can be made bearable if every small activity is not a constant reminder of the absence of their twin.

After the acute phase of grief is over, a child of school age should return to school, and his friends encouraged to invite him round so he does not get trapped by his own fears and lack of confidence. Children in middle childhood are not usually frightened by the idea of death and can sometimes appear quite callous.

Twins of all ages always have mixed feelings about each other, however close they may appear to be, and when they lose their twin, older twins may still need to be reassured that bad thoughts cannot hurt people. These worries may surface as nightmares which often bring an older child to a child and adolescent clinic.

Not only can parents idealize the lost twin, but the lone twin himself may idealize the lost companion of his infancy. He would have protected him, understood him, loved him. This can sometimes make it difficult for him to come to terms with life as it is, particularly if he is over- protected by his parents.

When a loved one dies, anger is sometimes directed towards the dead person – 'Why did they leave me? Why did they go away? A baby, a bringer of love, is often seen as an unacceptable object of anger, particularly by children, and more so if this has been a 'good' baby. So the family have to direct their anger elsewhere, perhaps towards each other, or perhaps, for a child, towards his friends and teachers at school.

Sometimes a lone twin, or an older brother or sister, becomes stuck with his angry feelings. If he has had to suppress his grief because his parents have been unable to talk about the death or were too overcome by grief themselves, his anger may not surface until later when it can be misunderstood. His feelings of anger against himself may make him push others away from him, feeling that he does not deserve their love, only punishment. Or he may unconsciously behave in such a way as to invite the punishment that he feels he deserves.

Not only does a bereaved child's behaviour sometimes change at school - a normally well behaved child becoming aggressive, or a normally happy outward-going child becoming withdrawn – but, as in adult grief, he may have great difficulty in concentrating. Daydreaming, tearfulness, not being able to answer simple questions, may all be part of the experience of loss, but should not give cause for concern. However, it is of the utmost importance that teachers are made aware of the situation, otherwise they may misinterpret the signs. Some children become temporary school refusers, fearful of who next may disappear from their world. Many children become clingy. Giving them the opportunity to talk is the best way to help them to grieve. This, and the security of a routine, enables them to work through their feelings.

All those who have lost a loved one know of the experience of constantly seeing the person on every street, but the identical twin may be haunted by his own reflection. Unlike the non-identical twin who, as he grows older, will leave his twin behind him in childhood, the identical twin may look in the mirror and say, 'This is how my brother would have looked if he were here now.'

Twins who have been bereaved as children may unconsciously always be looking for a partner to replace the lost brother or sister. Zazzo [2] tells us of a younger brother who lost one of a pair of older twin sisters. His sister was inconsolable and withdrew into her shell, until he willingly substituted himself for her lost twin. Parents who were bereaved of a twin in childhood may seek a twin in one of their own children of the same sex as their twin; even a grandmother may seek the lost twin in a grandchild.

Nothing can really prepare a twin for the loss, through death, of his partner. If the loss is in childhood, before separation has taken place, or in adulthood when a decision to stay together has been reached, then he has lost not only his twin but his twinness, his accepted place in society. There is a similarity to the situation of a widow whose status in her community has been totally dependent upon her husband. The sense, not only of loss, but of being lost, cannot be underestimated, and it may take the twin child or adult some time before he gains sufficient confidence to tackle life on his own.

It is important that parents and children share their grief. If a child feels that he should suppress his grieving because he must protect his parents, or if parents are unable to grieve so that the child may think that grieving is unacceptable, then it is likely to surface again in adolescence or later, when it may be much more damaging. Parents should not be in too much of a hurry to clear out a dead twin's belongings; it may be better to do this gradually and find out which of them has importance for the twin who is on his own.

When a twin is lost in adolescence, feelings from infancy and the work on separation and identity may remain unresolved. Parents should be aware that there may be a need to work through these feelings with professional help, although talking within the family, and with friends, can be a great healer.

A family that has come through a tragedy such as this will find that the bond between them has become closer and that they have strengths of which they were previously unaware.

Perhaps the most surprising fact is the importance both to the parents and the survivor that even if he lost his twin at birth, sometimes even before birth, he is still a twin. His co twin is an ever present reality.

~~~~~

## References:

1.  Bryan, E. (1983) *The nature and nurture of twins* London: Balliere Tindell

2.  Zazzo R. (1960) *Les Jumeaux-Le Couple et le Personne*. Paris: Presses Universitaires de France

# LYNNE SCHULZ

## HELPING MULTIPLE LOSS FAMILIES

*What began as a small organisation to cater for the needs
of any type of infant loss, has become a widely recognised
specialist in the field of multiple pregnancy loss.  Initially
I received approximately three enquiries per year, which
has grown to sometimes three a day.  E-mails come from all
around the world seeking information and support for twin
and higher order multiple pregnancy losses.  My books,
**The Diary** and **The Survivor** have become useful extensions
of the work that I do, allowing me access into the lives of
many individuals, and my website has given many families
and medical professionals access to information and support
groups that they were previously unable to find.*

~~~~~

Lynne Schulz is the Founder/Co-ordinator of Murraylands
Twin Loss, established in 1992, and based in Murray
Bridge, South Australia.  Lynne is a volunteer bereavement
counsellor and educator.   She is the author of the books,
*The Diary*, (inspired by her daughter Megan's life), and *The
Survivor,* (inspired by her son Rhys' life).

*Complete script of a speech presented at
the Lutherans For Life Convention, Christ Church Lutheran Church,
Murray Bridge, South Australia, on 9th October 2004.*
*© Lynne Schulz  2004*

# 4

## HELPING MULTIPLE LOSS FAMILIES

*Lynne Schulz*

The Murraylands Lutheran SISS (Stillborn Infant Support Service) was founded in October 1992 initially to bridge the gap between rural and city bereavement care services. Bereavement counselling at that time was basically non-existent and parents experiencing any form of infant loss were constantly being referred to Adelaide. What began as a small organisation to cater for the needs of any type of infant loss, has become a widely recognised specialist in the field of multiple pregnancy loss.

Initially I received approximately three enquiries per year, which has grown to sometimes three a day. E-mails come from all around the world seeking information and support for twin and higher order multiple pregnancy losses. My books, *The Diary*[1] and *The Survivor* [2] have become useful extensions of the work that I do, allowing me access into the lives of many individuals, and my website [3] has given many families and medical professionals access to information and support groups that they were previously unable to find.

In the beginning I was viewed as a threat by most of the larger bereavement care organisations throughout Australia, because I was seen to be encroaching on their territory and taking clients away from them. This was of course nonsense, however, I was determined to fight on to establish myself as a credible provider of twin loss bereavement care services throughout South Australia. Now, almost twelve years later, I think I am regarded as a useful colleague and am recognised around the world. Invitations to speak to groups where I was the only person in attendance, have now changed to full rooms of curious, enquiring minds.

It is good to see such a change in attitude towards the topic of infant loss that many people once feared and regarded as 'taboo' in everyday conversation. It is also good to see that other bereavement care organisations have learnt to work in with existing groups, in order to avoid the unnecessary doubling up of resources.

As with many things in life, not all goes according to plan, and there is one situation in particular which tends to haunt me whenever I am being introduced to an audience. Just before I gave a speech to a Lutheran Women's Guild meeting, the lady who was about to introduce me, turned and asked if I had something written down for her to read. Grabbing a copy of my book, *The Diary* I quickly pushed it towards her, pointed to the relevant section on the back cover, and told her to read it out.

All went smoothly until she reached the end and mispronounced one of the key words. Instead of telling people that I trained in "martial arts", she announced that I trained in "material arts". And to top it all off, the sea of puzzled faces looked none the wiser when I hastily jumped up and corrected her. So now I just tell everyone that I do karate!

## The importance of Bereavement Care

It is widely acknowledged throughout the world, that bereavement care is an important mental health issue, with far reaching ramifications throughout our society as a whole. Unresolved grief, or matters relating to death that are not properly handled can result in situations ranging from domestic violence, substance abuse, alcoholism, marriage breakdown, to extreme situations involving child abduction and even murder.

Our modern western society has made significant changes during the past decade in how it has handled singleton loss issues and no longer do parents hear cruel words such as, "Just go home and forget about it".

However, the same cannot be said for the treatment of multiple pregnancy loss families and it saddens me to continually hear stories from bereaved parents of how they were poorly treated by medical professionals, friends and family who simply did not understand. Harsh and unnecessary phrases such as, "Well at least you still have a baby", in situations relating to twin loss, still occur. If society has been slow to make improvements in its care of singleton loss families, it has been even slower to recognise and make similar improvements for multiple pregnancy loss families.

Where singleton loss families are encouraged to work through their grief and are offered various forms of memory creation to allow them to remember their precious babies, multiple loss families are often forgotten.

As I have mentioned in previous articles, families who raise a surviving twin or higher order multiple speak of having to live with a constant daily reminder of their loss. Survivors often speak of feeling isolated from the rest of the world; trying to understand why they feel different.

## The importance of educating about twin loss issues

In an effort to educate medical professionals, schools, government agencies, bereavement care organisations and church groups, the award-winning *Apex Australia Twin Loss Awareness Kit* [4] was created. As the mother of a surviving twin I have experienced ridicule and disbelief from friends, family, child carers and school teachers whenever I have even mentioned that my eldest son is a surviving twin, and therefore different to singleton children. In an attempt to make the lives of other twin loss families a little easier, myself and a small dedicated team set out to try and educate those who came into contact with multiple loss families such as my own to be a little more empathetic towards our unique needs.

Twinship evokes an enormous amount of curiosity and interest throughout our society. The media are often guilty of turning the whole topic of multiple births into a circus event. In my second book, *The Survivor,* I look at how twinship is viewed in different ways. Interestingly enough, the whole concept of twinship continues to be shrouded in mystical, magical, even romantic notions.

In explaining the differences between a singleton and multiple pregnancy, I want you to imagine that I am holding two apples. Each piece of fruit represents a pregnancy. The first apple is one complete unit, whilst the other has been sliced into two.

Even though one apple has been divided into portions, it remains exactly like the first one, i.e. one whole, healthy apple. Now, if we take away one half of the divided piece of fruit, what do we have left? We are left with part of an apple. It has not turned itself into a banana, or a grapefruit. It remains an apple.

When a baby dies in a twin pregnancy, it is like removing half of the apple. The picture now appears out of balance. It does not look quite right to the untrained eye. That is precisely how a surviving twin appears to the world – a slightly unbalanced picture. Something is missing and behavioural patterns and physical abilities may not be quite right. The child has not magically turned into a singleton package – that child will always be a twin for the rest of their entire life.

People who do not understand the concept of twin loss, and what it means to be a survivor, may become concerned at some of the apparently unusual behavioural traits that can be displayed. Sometimes those same people may suggest that the child requires special counselling or some other treatment. In actual fact, the child just needs someone with a 'trained eye' to view the picture in its correct perspective.

When our surviving twin Rhys was very young, he formed attachments with girls his own age, as if to subconsciously fill the void where his twin would have been. He also had a very annoying habit of 'tuning out' whenever we were talking to him. This would occasionally occur right in the middle of a conversation. Our family always referred to this as Rhys disappearing into 'Rhys-land'.

My son also displayed extremes in his motor skills, presenting a very unbalanced picture indeed. In his kindergarten years, it was noted that his fine motor skills, such as writing and drawing, were above average for a child his age, yet in comparison his gross motor skills, such as running and jumping, were far below average. He struggled to complete sporting activities and literally ran like a duck. We spent the first few years of his school life being constantly told by teachers that something was not quite right with our son, yet no one was able to provide a solution. My husband and I became angry and frustrated by the lack of interest from those around us in finding a solution. Eventually, we tried an activity where Rhys would have to work hard on perfecting both his fine and gross motor skills simultaneously. Something repetitive that would hopefully improve his abilities and not make him the subject of ridicule.

An opportunity arose to enrol him in a local karate academy so we decided to give it a try. During his early days at the martial arts academy he was considered by the instructor to be the least likely student to ever succeed. His co-ordination was absolutely atrocious and people would giggle at his efforts. However, Rhys was determined to prove himself, and now after many years of hard work, he is one of the best athletes in his class at high school, and is being groomed to eventually become a karate instructor. What I made mention of in *The Survivor* was that even though I would love to say to everyone, "go and get your child enrolled in a martial arts class", that would be unrealistic and quite irresponsible of me.

What I do say to parents is please do not give up in your search to find your answers, no matter how unconventional they may initially appear to be. Don't give up on your survivors because they do not give up on us!

When I was writing *The Survivor* I asked for input from mothers of surviving multiple birth children. Two stories which created a great deal of interest came from opposite ends of the globe. One was from a NSW mother of a surviving twin, whilst the other was from an American mother of two surviving triplets. Both spoke of unexplained happenings within their homes after their children had died. The woman in NSW told of toys moving for no apparent reason, and the lady in the US shared with me, a photo depicting a ghostly, angelic looking image that had appeared on the family's television set whilst the surviving two triplets sat in front of it for a family Christmas portrait.

When working on *The Survivor*, I finished the chapter entitled, "A Mother's Perspective" in the following manner in regards to my own situation with my deceased daughter, Megan.

*I feel her presence, even now after all these years. Is it just a wishful thought? Sometimes I turn around suddenly expecting to see someone standing behind me, but when I turn around, there is no one there.*

*Sometimes I feel that I am being watched by unseen eyes, but I am sitting in an empty room.*

Do our deceased children stay with us? Do they in turn watch over and protect us, hopefully from some of the horrors of the real world? I would like to think so. I will leave that thought with you.

Twin loss is a widespread issue which surpasses culture, language and distance. It occurs all too frequently right around the world. It is difficult to find enough supporting evidence regarding twin loss due to the fact that very little credible research has been carried out. Up until more recent times, unscrupulous people pertaining to be experts in multiple pregnancy loss issues have made things almost impossible in regards to getting the topic of twin loss taken seriously amongst the medical professional arena.

It does not help when some people lay claim that Vanishing Twin Syndrome for example, is the result of alien invasion, and if it wasn't such a tragic situation for many families around the world, it would be laughable.

It is not until you mention that famous people such as Elvis Presley was a surviving twin, that people in general begin to sit up and take more notice of what you are saying. And whenever the Holocaust is mentioned, the fact that twins were regarded as prized possessions receives even less acknowledgement. It was in the Auschwitz death camp during the mid forties, that Dr Josef Mengele particularly sought out twins for his cruel and sickening medical experiments. These ranged from injecting chemicals into children's eyes to see if they would change colour, to sewing a set of twins together to create his own conjoined twins.

Some cultures such as the Balinese and some Native American Indian tribes viewed deceased twins with fear, whilst other societies such as the Cameroon people of West Africa showed more respect.

British Psychotherapist Joan Woodward, author of the book, *The Lone Twin* [5] and founder of the Lone Twin Network based in England, [6] carried out extensive research into the opinions and emotions of adult surviving twins. She basically concluded that no matter what age the separation occurred, whether it be during birth or later in life, all twin loss is profound in its effect upon the survivors. Those survivors who were not told about their twinship and later discovered by accident, were able to find answers to questions that had haunted them for most of their lives. It enabled them to put their life into some type of perspective, allowing them to move forward in a more positive manner.

I have dealt with women who were told by well-meaning doctors, family and friends to keep the fact that they gave birth to twins a secret. This was in an ignorant, yet well-meaning attempt to avoid further pain, however unable to hold their secrets in, many years later, found little support from those around them. Some of these women have been placed in psychiatric care in an effort to allow them to finally acknowledge, grieve and come to terms with their tragic experiences.

In *The Survivor* emphasis is placed on the concept of honesty, by parents towards their surviving multiple birth children. Hiding the truth does not work, and asking people that we know to keep secrets for years on end, is both unfair and ridiculous. It is important that we acknowledge that by sharing the truth and being honest with our surviving twins, we can find a balance between a healthy reality and an unhealthy obsession.

Life has been interesting as a bereavement counsellor and educator. The organisation that trained me in counselling skills does not recognise me, yet many other authorities respect my opinion. I often refer to myself as a 'rebellious maverick;' but one of my NSW colleagues calls me a 'pioneer'. The media do not show much interest in my work, yet will promote people who have taken some of it and passed it off as their own. Thankfully I have received more 'thank yous' than threats but that is part of opening the door to people's private lives. Educating organisations in twin loss issues has seen personal counselling take a back seat at present. My current project is to distribute the remainder of the twin loss awareness kits throughout the state, and to prepare the nomination in order to take the whole project onto a national level.

If I have managed to open your minds to the whole concept of twin loss, and the more positive treatment of it, then I have succeeded here today. Kits are currently being used by Flinders Medical Centre to train their midwives, by the South Australia Police Blue Light State Council, by numerous hospitals, bereavement care groups, emergency services groups and schools. If what I have said today benefits just one family, then it was well worth it.

~~~~~

## References

1. Schulz, L.(1998) The Diary. Clever-Clogs Independent Publishers

2. Schulz, L.(2003) The Survivor. Pleasant Word 2003

3. The website adress is: http://lm.net.au/~schulz/siss/

4. For details contact Apex Club of Murray Bridge Inc., PO Box 132, Murray Bridge, South Australia 5253 Australia

5. Woodward, J (1998) The Lone Twin: understanding twin bereavement and loss. Free Association Books

6. The Lone Twin Network, PO Box 5653, Birmingham, B29 7JY England.

# ELIZABETH BRYAN

## THE DEATH OF A TWIN

*Death or disability is much more common in multiple
births than single children, especially in the perinatal
period. Parents face particular problems in that their loss
may be underestimated; their grieving may be impeded
by the confusion between the live and the dead baby, and
the constant reminder in the survivor may be painful. The
surviving twin often suffers profoundly from the loss and
may need lifelong support. The value of the twinship should
always be respected.*

~~~~~

Elizabeth Bryan is a paediatrician, an international expert on
multiple births and past President of the ISTS (International
Society for Twin Studies). She was founder and first director
of the Multiple Births Foundation, an independent charity
based at Queen Charlotte's & Chelsea Hospital in West
London, which is an international authority on the care,
development and special problems of children born as twins,
triplets or more. Dr Bryan was a co-founder of TAMBA (the
Twins and Multiple Births Association, a UK based charity).
She has also written books on twins and edited a Special
Issue of Twin Research on The Loss of a Twin or Triplet.

*Palliative Medicine, 1995 Jul; 9 (3): 187-92.*
*Entire article reproduced with permission of author and
by permission of Sage Pubications Ltd.*

# 5

## THE DEATH OF A TWIN

*Elizabeth Bryan*

### Introduction

Many more parents of twins have to face the tragedy of
bereavement than those with singletons since the mortality
rate of twins is much higher from the time of conception.
Very many more twins are conceived than delivered, more
even than until recently thought. A twin pregnancy is
very often not detected, so the total numbers lost in early
pregnancy are unknown. Later, the risk of a stillbirth is over
twice that for singletons and mortality is five times higher in
the neonatal period.[1] This increased risk of death persists,
if at lower levels, through at least the first year of life. The
incidence of sudden infant death syndrome (SIDS) amongst
twins is higher, probably partly due to the adverse factors
known to be associated with both twinning and SIDS, such
as prematurity and low birth weight.[2] For the most part, and
not surprisingly, the death of a twin will have the same sort
of effect on other members of the family as the death of any
other child.

Parents who lose both their twins suffer a plain,
and conspicuous, tragedy. Yet they will also receive the
unqualified sympathy of relatives, friends and the medical
profession. The position of parents who lose one twin
is not nearly so simple. There are some aspects of the
bereavement, both for the parents and for the surviving
twin, which are special, particularly where one twin is
stillborn or has died within the first few days. For deaths
that occur beyond the neonatal period, the survivor will

51

never have known life without a (mostly constant) partner and find this deeply disturbing. The parents' loss too is often underestimated.

## Death in the perinatal period

In a society where death is still largely a taboo subject, the birth of a dead baby is perhaps the hardest of all to acknowledge. Professionals try to ignore or even forget what has happened.[3] People manage to move on distressingly quickly (for the parents), even when it is a single baby who has died. When a twin baby dies at birth or during the early weeks, this reality-avoidance can be accomplished with even greater ease. Attention and emotions focus on the surviving child and the parents are too often encouraged to follow this example. They are not allowed space to grieve. Too often they are made to feel guilty by misguided remarks such as, 'How lucky that you still have one healthy baby' or 'Two babies would have been such a handful.'

The mother especially will be confused by the contradiction in her feelings as she simultaneously rejoices in the new life and grieves for the death of the other. It is only by allowing, indeed encouraging, a mother to think and talk about her dead baby that the normal mourning process can take place and she can be released to give her full love to the survivor.[4] If a mother is forced to concentrate on the healthy child to the exclusion of the dead baby, she may start idealizing the latter and positively alienate herself from the survivor. Its normal crying, feeding behavior or restlessness may irritate her quite unreasonably. She may feel it is punishing her. Child abuse would not be unexpected in situations of this kind and has been reported in a surviving twin of a 'cot death.'[5]

To facilitate her mourning the mother needs clearly to distinguish the two babies in her mind. This can be helped by assembling or creating substantive memories of the dead baby. Having seen and handled the baby will greatly help her to recognize it as a person in its own right. Photographs should always be taken, preferably of the two babies together, even if the parents show little interest in these at the time. If the opportunity is missed, a photographic department can usually merge two separate photographs later. Some artists are prepared to make attractive sketches using the original photographs. This will be the most appropriate where one baby has died some time before delivery. Many people need to have a memorable funeral for their baby and an individual grave or memorial. Even if stillborn, it is especially wise for the baby to be given a name, not least so that the survivor can easily refer to their twin in later life.[6]

When both babies are born alive but one is likely to die soon, from gross malformations or severe birth anoxia for example, parents should be encouraged to give their time to the ill baby. Parents want to do as much as possible for their sick baby while they can. This will reduce any guilt they may feel about the twin's death and provide extra memories for them to treasure over the years.

## Death in childhood

In childhood, twins are little if any more likely to die than singletons, but for those who do - be it from an accident, chronic illness or acute infection - the effects on the survivor can be devastating.[7] These effects are of course greater when the twins have had little experience of being separated or when the one who died was the 'leader'. For such survivors, the belief of some African tribes may appear frighteningly apt, that the spirit of the dead twin must be preserved in order to ensure the wholeness of the survivor.[8] Single surviving Yoruba twins from Nigeria carry a wooden image representing their dead twin around their neck or waist, which is said to give at once company to the survivor and refuge for the spirit of his or her dead twin.

People who are not twins rarely recognize how intimate and constant is the twin-twin relationship. They see much more of each other than of either parent. Their relationships with others, even with the mother, are essentially triadic. They even very often create their own language. The loss of this partner can be as profound as the loss of any other partner.

The healthy twin should therefore be as closely involved with the brother or sister's illness and death as their level of understanding allows. Only so can they be adequately prepared for life without a previously constant partner. At the same time, the twin may need reassuring that he or she will not also succumb to the same illness, or indeed, will not also die. Euphemistic substitutes for the word 'death', such as 'long sleep' can lead to the survivor fearing sleep, and 'loss' may precipitate anger about the parents' carelessness.

The unknown and unseen are often more incomprehensible and frightening than reality. For a twin that can be especially relevant. There are advantages, both to the chronically ill child and the healthy twin, in being together through the final weeks. The paediatrician, Janet Goodall and the parents of a terminally ill five-year-old have sensitively and revealingly described how they coped at home rather than in hospital. This enabled both older and younger sisters to come to terms with the death of their brother much more easily then they would have done if they had been excluded from the whole experience.[9] When the brother died, the image employed by the parents was that of moving house. His body, the house, was no longer needed now he had moved to a new home. This image may help families who are uncomfortable with the concept of heaven as the new home. There are also books such as *Waterbugs and dragonflies*,[10] which can help children to understand the concept of moving to a new but unseen life; waterbugs are unable to see or imagine the dragonflies they are soon to become.

If the ill child has to be admitted to hospital, there will be times when the twin should accompany them not only for their mutual comfort but for the mother's practical convenience. One mother described how she had to stop breastfeeding when one of her babies went into hospital with pyloric stenosis and she was refused permission to bring the twin in with her. It can be extremely painful for both twins when the stress of illness in hospital causes their first experience of separation. Even those children who are used to being separated will often get great comfort from each other's presence at such a time. It is hard to convince some hospital authorities how important it is to allow twins to be admitted together.

It is also necessary to respect each child's need for individual attention. Plainly there will be times when the ill child will want the parents to herself or himself, especially when the illness is a long one. The healthy child may suffer even more from the parents' lack of attention or that of other people. Not only do well-meaning friends naturally tend to focus on the ill child, but this one also acquires a lot of 'special friends' in the doctors, therapists and nurses. The healthy child's needs must therefore be carefully attended to and some 'special friends' designated whose role is to give them some extra attention at a painful and puzzling time. This may also help to avoid the jealously and guilt that these children often suffer.

**The surviving twin**

The number of single surviving twins in the UK is difficult to determine, but estimated range between 5% and 15% of all twin pairs.[11] The price of being a single survivor may be very high. Some of the surviving twin's characteristic problems, both in relation to their parents and themselves, are discussed below, but many are still ill understood.

Even those twins who appear psychologically and socially unscathed may suffer silently and profoundly from their bereavement. Too often their dead twin is never mentioned. It is rare, for instance, for a teacher at school, or even in a playgroup, to know of a twin who died at birth or soon after. Yet the child's first drawings may show that he needs to express than twinship. Perhaps there is the recurring second figure. One three-year-old, whose twin was stillborn, was repeatedly attracted to depleted objects: the toy car without a wheel, the doll missing an arm.[12]

For a twin, the constant reminder in themselves of their twin may be deeply painful. The daily shave for a young man may be an agonizing vision of his twin. One factor may be that the survivor not only has survivor guilt but has a terrible feeling of vulnerability and of the seemingly arbitrary nature of survival.

Through the work of Joan Woodward, a psychotherapist in Birmingham, whose own identical twin died in early childhood, we have learned much about the profound and unique sense of loss felt by many adult single surviving twins. By interviewing over 200 bereaved twins, including many who had lost their twin at birth or in infancy, this special kind of loss is now better understood.[13] Some survivors feel their parents blame them for a newborn twin's death. Some have been told stories that seem cruel. One was told that she had 'taken her brother's food' and another that her sister had died because she 'had been starved and finally kicked out by me'.

When a twin dies, the survivor may well feel guilty about being the one chosen to live. This guilt, of course, is compounded if they come to think they were directly or indirectly responsible for the twin's death. Guilt will clearly be reinforced by parents who might seem to have preferred the other child to live. It is all too easy to idealize the dead child and forget that they too would sometimes have been lazy, untidy or generally irritating. Single survivors will also feel the more inadequate if their parents have placed undue store on being 'parents of twins' - as many do - and too obviously betray this aspect of their grief.

The dying child may have outstanding business to settle before he dies, such as deciding to whom his special possessions should go. This is natural, but the survivor should likewise be involved in the process of sorting out the twin's belongings after death. One mother described how, after the accidental death of one of her 14-year-old identical twin sons, his brother preserved the twin's part of the bedroom tidily for many months. Gradually, however, there were stages of replacement and finally he decided which of the possessions should become his own and which should be given away. He then took over the whole room for himself, keeping just one shelf of his brother's treasures. It is worth noting that this same boy was distressed to find when he returned from school (some months after the accident in which he too had been injured) to find all signs of his twin had been removed from the school and that he had not even been involved in the reallocation of his brother's coat hook. As the months passed, this bereaved teenager also assumed some of his brother's qualities. Having been the less responsible and tidy of the two, he became increasingly dependable and orderly. Several adult twins, notably Norris McWhirter,[14] whose twin brother was murdered, have described how twinship had enhanced the performance of both (the pacer and runner effect), but that after death the choice seems to be either to exist painfully as half a person or take on the strength of both.

After death, the parents will have to decide whether
the twin should see the dead sibling and whether the child
should attend the funeral. This must be the personal decision
of the parents, but even a young child may clearly express
its own wishes. For many children it can be reassuring to
see how peaceful their brother or sister looks after they have
died; they might otherwise harbour horrifying images. Some
children may like to help prepare the coffin. One 9-year-
old, whose brother had died of leukaemia, took a long time
carefully arranging the football boots, cap and football in the
coffin.

Young children have great difficulty in understanding
death's finality that their twin will never return.[15] One three-
year-old, whose brother had died in hospital six months
earlier, insisted on taking some of his toys to the doctor at
Christmas time, so that they could be given to his twin.
Many parents, whilst still grieving themselves, find the
disturbed behavior of the survivor particularly distressing.
One two-and-a-half-year-old suddenly lost his monozygotic
twin brother from bacterial meningitis. Having had normal
speech development as well as their own elaborate 'twin
language' he became silent. Six weeks later his mother
took him to the mirror to point out some dirty marks on his
face. His expression lit up for a few seconds only to turn to
anguish as he realized the reflection was his own, not that of
his twin. He refused to go near a mirror again and became
increasingly withdrawn and destructive. There may be
profound psychic injuries that do not show any immediate
overt symptoms, so that the closest attention to, and
reassurance, of the surviving twin may be crucial.

Some children's behavior at these times can be so
difficult as to disrupt family life, and parents may well
disagree profoundly - in complete good faith- on the best
methods of helping their unhappy child. Marital discord
over this is common. All families should therefore be

offered support and bereavement counselling from the earliest possible stage in the hope of preventing or reducing both the child's difficulties and the family's tensions.

A child whose twin has died in the perinatal period may later feel distress, anxiety or just curiosity about it. They should feel free to talk about these feelings and not suppress them because they expect talking about the dead sibling to upset their parents. If their fear is actually justified, it is crucial that there should be someone else with whom they may comfortably talk about the twin. I have met many adult twins who were quite unable to talk to their parents about the death of their twin. Others find profound relief when finally they are able to do so. One surviving twin talked to her mother for the first time about her stillborn brother 22 years later. It was a relief to them both and led to them holding a memorial service at the unmarked grave.

I believe all single surviving twins should hear about their twinship, preferably from the start, and be encouraged to ask questions and express their feelings, whether considered rational or not. Some feel angry: angry with the twin for deserting them; angry for causing such unhappiness in the family; angry for making them, the survivor, feel guilty. They may also feel anger towards their parents for 'allowing' the twin to die.

Reactions are unpredictable. One mother waited seven years before she, with great trepidation, told her son of his stillborn twin. The child's reaction astonished her: he was elated by the news of his special status. The next day he rushed into school to tell his teacher and friends that, 'I was a twin.' Many twins will treasure mementoes of their dead twin and some will enjoy making their own scrapbook or collection of mementoes. They may add their own drawings. One of the frequent confusions for both the parents and the surviving twin is at what age to picture the lost one.

Other surviving twins will have more complex feelings. Some have secret fantasies, which can be frightening. One five-year-old's life was being seriously curbed by the ghost of his twin. He feared to go upstairs on his own and was unable to put his hand out from under the blankets to get a drink for fear of the ghost. It was only by talking about and drawing these fears that he was gradually helped to come to terms with them and to accept that the ghost would do him no harm. Indeed he came to think of the ghost as a friend.

## Parents' attitude to the surviving twin

Most mothers have ambivalent feelings towards the surviving twin. Some over-protect the survivor, others reject them; many do both. They are thankful to have this baby (or child) to love, yet also feel that this child is in some way responsible for the death of the other. Did the survivor take an unfair share of the intrauterine nutrition? With an older child, the mother may feel that the accident that killed one was somehow the fault of the other. Sometimes, of course, this is true.

Many parents are haunted by the vision of their dead child in the living twin. One mother dreaded washing her two-year-old's hair because when his hair was wet he looked most like his dead brother. Another mother described how her 18-month-old daughter acquired a number of mannerisms that had once been peculiar to the dead twin.

Such ever present reminders of the lost child can be so painful that the mother may temporarily reject the twin and give an unfair amount of attention to other siblings. This problem may even arise with a stillborn baby. One mother who had never seen the stillborn baby found that each time she looked at his live twin she was unable to stop herself wondering what the dead one was like.

Fathers of twins may be especially affected by the death of a twin baby or child as, by force of circumstances, they are likely to have been more involved than with the singleton right from the start. They are also sometimes less used to expressing or discussing their feelings and therefore cope with their loss much less easily than the mother. Both parents will need a lot of support in coping with the other's grief and with the reactions of the surviving twin.

Most fathers are extremely proud of having twins and unfortunately some, in the early years, persist in thinking of them as a single unit. The destruction of this unit may therefore leave an incomplete child, one whom the father may reject. After the loss of a two-year-old twin son, one father insisted on the removal of all photographs of the pair. As the twins had never been photographed separately this meant removing all photographs of the live twin too. He was able to give his love and attention to the five-year-old sister but wanted nothing to do with the surviving twin, who was too painful a reminder of the lost son, and the lost twinship.

## Conclusions

The death of a child is devastating for any family and particular problems exist when this child is a twin. Attention may be focused on the surviving twin such that it prevents adequate opportunities for grief on the part of the parents, the surviving twin and other family members.

Most parents continue to think of their single surviving child as a twin even if the other was stillborn, and they like other people to do the same. For this reason some parents who have lost a twin continue to join in the activities of their local twins club and this is generally well understood by the other parents. Other bereaved parents not surprisingly find contact with twins or their parents too painful. They may however welcome an opportunity to share their feelings with other bereaved parents, particularly those who have had twins.

The Twins and Multiple Births Association Bereavement Support Group can provide such contacts individually or via their newsletter. This group also holds three-monthly lunchtime meetings at Queen Charlotte's and Chelsea Hospital in London, where the Multiple Births Foundation offers professional support and a specialized bereavement clinic to parents, bereaved children and bereaved adults. The Multiple Births Foundation also puts bereaved adult twins in touch with other such adults through the Lone Twin Network. Contact addresses for these organizations are given in the Appendix.

## References

1. Botting B, Macdonald-Davis I, Macfarlane A. (1987) Recent trends in the incidence of multiple births and their mortality. *Arch.Dis Child* 62: 941-50

2. Beal S. (1983) *Some epidemiological factors about sudden death syndrome (SIDS) in South Australia.* In: Tildon JT, Roeder LM, Steinschneider A eds. *Sudden infant death syndrome.* New York; Academic Press pp.15-28

3. Bourne S. (1968) The psychological effects of stillbirths in women and their doctors *JR Coll Gen Pract*16:103-12

4. Lewis E. (1979) Mourning by the family after a stillbirth or neonatal death. *Arch Dis Child* 1979; 54:303-306

5. Bluglass K. (1980) Psychiatric morbidity after cot death. *Practitioner* 224:533-39.

6. Lewis E, Bryan E. (1988) Management of perinatal loss of a twin. *Br Med J* 297:1321-23.

7. Bernabei P, Levi G. (1976) Psychopathological problems in twins during childhood. *Acta Genet Med Gemellol (Roma)* 25: 381-83.

8. Elniski J. (1994) Finding one's twin. *Parabola* 19:47-51.

9. Cotton M, Cotton G, Goodhall J. (1981) A brother dies at home. *Matern Child Health* 6:288-92.

10. Sticknet D. (1982) *Waterbugs and dragonflies*. London: Mowbray.

11. Bryan EM. (1992) *Twins and higher multiple births: a guide to their nature and nurture*. Sevenoaks: Edwards Arnold.

12. Lewis E. (1983) *Stillbirths: Psychological consequences and strategies of management*. In: Mulinsky A, Freidman EA, Gluck I eds. *Advances in prenatal medicine* 3. New York: Plenum, pp.203-45.

13. Woodward J. The bereaved twin. *Acta Genet Med Gemello (Roma)* 1988; 37:173-80.

14. McWhirter N. Ross (1976) *The story of a shared life*. London: Churchill Press.

15. Goodhall J. (1994) *Thinking like a child about death and dying*. In: Hill L ed. *Caring for dying children and their families*. London: Chapman and Hall, pp. 16-31.

## Appendix

**The Multiple Births Foundation**, Hammersmith House Level 4, Queen Charlotte's & Chelsea Hospital, Du Cane Road, London, W12 0HS.
Telephone: 0208 383 3519
E-mail: info@multiplebirths.org.uk
*(Please note: the bereavement clinic is no longer operational.)*

**TAMBA Bereavement Support Group**
2, The Willows, Gardner Road, Guildford, Surrey GU1 4PG
Telephone: 0870 770 3305
Website: www.tamba-bsg.org.uk

**Lone Twin Network**
P.O. Box 5653, Birmingham, B29 7JY

# CAROLYN MAY DAWN PHD

## THE SURVIVING TWIN: PSYCHOLOGICAL, EMOTIONAL, AND SPIRITUAL IMPACTS OF HAVING EXPERIENCED A DEATH BEFORE OR AT BIRTH.

*For my doctoral dissertation I investigated the psychological, emotional and spiritual effects in later life of twin loss that occurred in utero or at birth. This research sought to uncover feelings, attitudes, life problems and behaviour problems from the perspective of the surviving twin. Here are some of my later reflections on that study.*

~~~~~

Dr. Carolyn M. Dawn is an educator in both secondary education and transpersonal psychology. She received a Master's Degree in Education from Stanford University and completed her doctorate at the Institute of Transpersonal Psychology in Palo Alto, CA, USA. She currently works with adolescents and also serves as a grief counselor and consultant to individuals, organizations, and community. She is herself a surviving twin.

*Original article based on a doctoral dissertation of the same title and completed in 2003 for The Institute of Transpersonal Psychology, Palo Alto, California, USA.*

# 6

## THE SURVIVING TWIN: PSYCHOLOGICAL, EMOTIONAL, AND SPIRITUAL IMPACTS OF HAVING EXPERIENCED A DEATH BEFORE OR AT BIRTH.

*Carolyn May Dawn, Ph.D.*

### Overview

For my doctoral dissertation, this research, concluded in 2003, collected quantitative and qualitative data from 51 surviving adult twins, 39 women and 12 men, who had lost a twin either in utero, during birth, or within the first three days of life. The population sample desired was voluntarily self-identified surviving twins who either sought support and communication with others or expressed interest specifically regarding this situation. Forty-one of the 51 participants (80%) were drawn from the Twinless Twins International support group and 10 from referrals. As stated in their brochure, "Twinless Twins Support Group International was founded for one single purpose: to serve in support of twins (all multiple births) who suffer from the loss of companionship of their twin."[1] I was hoping for a deliberately biased sample in order to explore the issues, reactions, feelings, problems, questions, healing, treatments, and the entire realm that they themselves discovered and experienced.

The study was not intended to prove or disprove prenatal memory or its possible influence; it was intended to research the emerging anecdotal reports of surviving twins' psychological, emotional, and spiritual experiences with regard to the death of their co-twin.

The basic research design was a self-administered questionnaire including short answer demographic data, Likert scales, and write-in questions that were exploratory and open-ended in structure. Quantitative data from 15 Likert scales were crosstabulated with circumstances of when the co-twin died, the cause of death, and the age at which the survivor learned of the loss. The qualitative data were analyzed with rigorous content analysis.

## Major Findings: Support and Validation

Qualitative content analysis from the written questionnaires produced five major themes:

(a) Surviving twins felt lonely and guilty
(b) They had difficulty with intimate relationships, attachment and bonding
(c) They often longed for a special kind of closeness that remained elusive and unattainable
(d) They strongly felt information about their twinship should have been given freely and talked about early in life
(e) They thrived on emotional support for their loss and suffered from the lack of it.

Support and validation emerged as one of the major findings of this study. The initial research question was, What were the effects of support or nonsupport and validation by others? Results of the circumstances of death revealed quantitative data suggesting that lack of information and support resulted in the surviving twin suffering more severe negative consequences, and that those less resourced were not able to deal with the consequences in a positive and healing way. Both at birth and later in life, experiencing connection and validation was reported as crucial.

First, getting accurate and truthful information, being made aware of their twinship, was deemed essential. The participants pleaded for open discussions and thrived better when this was done early in life. They wanted to talk about it; they were emphatic about this. Again, from the results it appeared that without validation and acknowledgment of the truth, including the inner truth within oneself, there was suffering. The findings of this study reinforced a general psychological truth that grief and loss often stimulate a search for meaning. Frankl[2], writing about his experiences of surviving the Nazi concentration camps, perceived that in order to maintain the will to live, the prisoners had to search for some larger purpose for their suffering. His development of logotherapy was based on humanity's deepest longing, he believed—to find meaning. So too these surviving twins expressed a need to come to terms with many of the existential questions their loss gave rise to.

**Implications and Possible Practical Applications**

The results of the study indicated that surviving twins who are not aware of their twinship or who have very little validation and support for having lost a twin while in the womb or at birth may be adversely affected emotionally, psychologically and spiritually. It was further shown that negative effects are ameliorated with direct, open communication from the beginning from parents and society, including medical personnel. Obstetricians, nurses, pediatricians and all who work with maternal and fetal care were entreated by these participants to be apprised of the impact such a death may have on the survivor and to act accordingly to alleviate possible guilt, inexplicable loneliness, and self-recrimination. This appeared to be a situation where early detection and early treatment might save a lifetime of anguish and despair. Results so far produced by this and other research are consistent: tell them, tell them early, validate their experience.

These issues may involve 15% of our population.[3, 4, 5] The question might be raised, as technological birth advances, is difficulty in maintaining secure intimate relationships concomitantly being impaired? It would seem advisable to err in the direction of caution, as evidence is mounting that these surviving twins do "remember" and are affected. The twins' reports, as well as the findings, reflected that training is necessary to alert the scientific and medical personnel that there is a practical and social value to be gained from honoring cellular knowing and by assuming the experiences of the infant at birth have been imprinted in this cellular if not intuitive level and may manifest psychologically and emotionally in the personality that develops and infiltrates our society.

Findings in the area of bonding and attachment may also have important implications. Where did the feelings of loss and something missing come from? Sometimes, the parents had not even spoken of it, and sometimes the individual did not know he/she was a twin until adulthood. Woodward[6] maintained that the parents' attitude most affected future relationships, deferring to Bowlby's attachment theory. However, in the case of twin loss, a new model of attachment theory may be indicated based on *the attachment being to the primary or earliest partner, the twin.*

The emotional dynamics of attachment theory may therefore be applied but reinterpreted. Bowlby[7] asserted that the bond of love formed and maintained in early attachment is experienced as grief when severed. However, the attachment bond endures, and the various forms of behavior instinctual in the human to elicit renewal of the bond may require physical contact or actively seeking reassurance from the attachment figure. From this perspective, it is not difficult to see how failure to recognize the surviving twin's distress would result in an inability to return to equilibrium. Bowlby[8] described this as a phase of protest characterized by both physiological and psychological distress. If the bond is not restored, the effort wanes but not the need. The person's behavior is in a perpetual state of chronic distress.[9] He compares the loss of a loved person to be no less traumatic psychologically than a severe wound is physiologically. Similarly, the process of mourning may be compared to physical healing: it takes time and may lead eventually to the ability to make and maintain love relationships, or may take a course that leads to impaired function in the area of love relationships.[10]

Thus, the difficulties surviving twins might have in intimate relationships. It seems they had bonded in utero, and the loss was not of the parent but of the relationship with the twin. This is the perspective of prenatal psychology, that there is a felt sense of the twin in utero, that the loss is experienced. This has enormous implications in a practical and immediate way, for birthing methods and attitudes may need to be adjusted. Furthermore, in a wider context, one may question whether the current mainstream body of knowledge fails to deliver the information and support that surviving multiples need. Only those families that naturally allowed the twin to be part of the family spared the twins in this study from searching for freedom from grief and loneliness. If the underlying principles are about support and mirroring, this study may provide evidence to support or suggest that the prenatal or perinatal issues of loss may be generalized to other types of situations.

## Conclusion

Analysis of the data clearly showed that surviving twins were lonely, felt something was missing, felt guilty, and

had difficulty in maintaining intimate relationships, just as
the anecdotal reports showed. However this study showed
something more. It revealed that the actual circumstances
of the death, the causes, and the age at which they found
out were not the most significant factors in determining
whether they were distressed. What did matter was whether
their internal truth was seen, whether they were heard, and
whether they were validated in this highly intuitive and inner
sense of loss and grief and longing. What mattered more
was how the parents dealt with the circumstances, not what
the circumstances were.

Some were not told at all but overheard conversations
or found out by mistake. The anecdotal reports and The
Lone Twin Study[11] concluded that the death of the twin at
birth negatively affects parent/child bonding. This was not
strictly supported by the findings of this study. The median
for good relationship with mother was high, and bonding
occurred oftentimes even when the twin reported a great
sense of incompleteness and loneliness. It was not that
they didn't bond, necessarily. Profiles can be delineated, all
pointing to the same conclusion. First, there were those who
bonded well, were supported, whose lives were working, and
who either felt spiritually connected to the twin or accepted
the loneliness. Second were those who received little or
no support, were more depressed, and were unable to form
fulfilling relationships when acknowledgment at birth was
not there and when later in life open discussion was not
available either.

The crucial factors were twofold: how the death was
dealt with at the time by the parents and others involved,
and how the issue was dealt with subsequently, whether
others were present to the reality that a tragic death and
loss occurred. Not to recognize this was to invalidate the
internal experience of the twin, regardless of the maturity

of the thinking mind. That seems to confirm other prenatal research and theory that early experience is felt and known on a somatic level.

The bottom line is that what really mattered was being validated and supported in one's own truth and having one's own truth be honored, regardless of what the other person's opinion was. The surviving twins needed to be allowed to be in touch with themselves and to be honored as human beings. This emerged from the data in that those who were, to the extent they were, did not have as many difficulties with the same issues as those who were not. It was not, then, the death of the twin that made the difference.

In addition, almost unanimously the cry was to have this issue be openly talked about right from the beginning. The survivors fervently gave suggestions and advice:

- Give information truthfully, and allow feelings to be expressed.
- Encourage openness of communication.
- Educate the medical profession.
- Teach the parents how to deal with the survivor
- Educate the public that this lost twin is a real force.

No less than the connection between twins reared apart, there is mounting evidence that the connection engendered from being a multiple is not destroyed if the separation was through death.

As for relationships and bonding, both the quantitive and qualitative findings revealed that the twins in this study often bonded well with both parents, and though supported and validated, they could still feel lonely, incomplete or a great sense of loss or of something missing. Some twins in this study had found ameliorating factors, and others had not. Religious belief, though deemed important, was not as frequently reported as support and validation from humans!

It seems clear to these participants that when their
co-twin died, he or she suffered the loss of a bond that began
in utero, and when it was unrecognized, the loss could not be
grieved and the wound could not be healed. The results they
reported were severe difficulties and impairments in future
adult relationships. When the bond was recognized they
fared much better, whether that was initiated by the parents
or later in counseling, by friends or supporting others, or by
turning it over to God.

## Author's Comments

The seeds of this research study were sown in my own birth
story, which surfaced over a 30-year period in adulthood.
Gradually, disturbing sensing memories of having had a
traumatic birth and extreme anxiety in the first two months
or so of infancy became stronger and stronger. For these
I was unable to find any source within traditional or even
transpersonal psychology and psychotherapy. Awareness
came to me through dreams, hypnosis, altered states, and in
age regression processes: In the womb there was another,
who withered away as I flourished. Later, I had a lucid
dream in which there was a terror just before my birth, as I
was about to be born. I woke myself up, but only to reenter
the dream and experience again that first ecstatic breath,
which empowered me. But the discomforts grew. I began to
develop a fear of not being able to breathe and also a feeling
that death was imminent, physically. Finally, I reported all
this to my mother, who naively remarked, "Oh, didn't I ever
tell you that you were part of a twin?" She hadn't. I seemed
to carry the body memories of panic to survive, which I
experienced, I suppose, as a generalized anxiety. Could I
have been born not only terrified but grieving? Because
this emerged in my own experience, I wanted to discover if
other twins who survived when their co-twin did not would

report similar issues. I was fascinated by the possibilities of discovering the lifelong effects of such twin loss. It was my belief and experience at the time that these influences might be a significant source of personality development and that these imprints might set an underlying pattern for all future relationship and belief systems.

In evaluating the results of this study, it is important to be cognizant, however, of several considerations. First, the research participants were a deliberately biased sample. The information garnered from these participants did not represent twins who had the same situation in their lives but did not join a support group.

Second, attributing cause and effect is always problematic. Is one grieving because one has lost a loved one, or are other factors at play? Also, the nature of this specific material may be elusive, as it concerns an event that took place prenatally or at birth, a time about which there is little definitive scientific, psychological, theoretical, philosophical, or spiritual agreement. Furthermore, dysfunctional family relationships, physical effects of birth events, social and economic influences on the family, and a myriad of other developmental factors may be intertwined with the reported effects of twin loss.

Third, talk shows and mass media publicizing of twin loss may have exerted some influence in general public awareness, possibly influencing the respondents. Many reported reading articles, watching a television program, and finding information and recommended reading on the Internet.

Finally, and most important, before definitive interpretations may be made, a control group is necessary to assess whether surviving twins have been more affected by any negative birth experience than others who did not lose a twin.

## References for this extract:

1. Twinless Twins International. (1993). *Twinless Twins Support Group International* [Brochure]. Fort Wayne, IN: Raymond Brandt, Ph.D., Ed.D.

2. Frankl, V. (1984). *Man's search for meaning* (Rev. ed.). New York: Simon & Schuster. (Original work published 1959)

3. Boklage, C. E. (1995). *The frequency and survival probability of natural twin conceptions.* In L. Keith, E. Papiernik, D. Keith, & B. Luke (Eds.), *Multiple pregnancy: Epidemiology, gestation & perinatal outcome* (pp. 41-50). New York: Parthenon.

4. Botting, B., Macdonald-Davis, I., & Macfarlane, A. (1987). Recent trends in the incidence of multiple births and their mortality. *Arch Dis Child,* 62, 941-950.

5. Keith, L., Papiernik, E., Keith, D., & Luke, B. (Eds.). (1995). *Multiple pregnancy: Epidemiology, gestation & perinatal outcome.* New York: Parthenon.

6. Woodward, J. (1988). The bereaved twin. *Acta Genet Med Gemellol Roma,* 37(2), 173-180.

7. Bowlby, J. (1980). *Loss, sadness and depression.* London: Penguin.

8. Ibid., p. 41.

9. Ibid., p. 42

10. Ibid., p. 43.

11. Woodward, J. (1988) op.cit.

# WRETCHED

While walking down the street the other day
It struck me that my life had all but slipped away
They struck me right between the eyes
Those living lies

For I was dead and shrunken, grey and small
Disguised as an india-rubber ball
Disguised,   a fake

And the spirit sang in the tree
But not in me

Could I take life roughly in my grasp
Pull it here and there against its will
I am so still
I would command    say life thou wilt return
unto me    unto me   who's he?
Or could I twist myself about
To make a hole
This shammy leather   my desert
This weightless leaden shape

To let the water in
To fill with life, with life again
Amen   Amen

*Nick Owen*

~~~~~

*This was written in 1970, in my first year at university.
I was going though a period of existential death, when I saw
the world through the eyes of my dead twin, but at the time
I did not realise it.*

© Nick Owen 1970

# JOAN WOODWARD & BRYONY GOODE

## A WOMAN IN HER THIRTIES WHO LOST AN IDENTICAL SISTER AT BIRTH

*Bryony Goode's identical twin sister was stillborn but it was not until adulthood that she realised the profound impact of this loss. She joined the Lone Twin Network and began the process of reclaiming her twin.*

~~~~

Joan Woodward is a psychotherapist. In 1982 she decided to look into the consequences of death amongst twins. She founded the Lone Twin Network (originally called the Lone Twin Register) in May 1989 to offer a network of contacts and support to anyone whose twin has died, at whatever stage of life.

Bryony Goode was a teacher for 19 years before the birth of her son in 2005. As a member of the Lone Twin Network, she contributed her story to Joan Woodward's book, *The Lone Twin: understanding twin bereavement and loss.* This story has been selected from among many similar stories in this book, written by lone twins themselves.

# 7

## A WOMAN IN HER THIRTIES WHO LOST AN IDENTICAL SISTER AT BIRTH

I cannot remember a time when I did not know I was an identical twin. My family have always talked about it, in what seemed to me a detached way. By that, I mean that it has always been discussed as an interesting fact, but not as something which could have affected me very much, although my parents thought that my continual crying as a baby might be to do with me missing my twin. I myself did not connect my feelings and experiences to losing my sister before birth until I was in my late twenties.

My mother did not know that she had been expecting twins until after we were born and neither did the hospital staff. The first hint that it was not a straightforward labour was when my mother was told that there was a 'soft head', but the hospital staff would not explain what that meant. After twenty-two hours, they removed my stillborn sister. I was then delivered with forceps as I was becoming exhausted. I weighed 4 lb 11 oz and my sister weighed 4 lb 10 oz. I was in the special baby unit for three weeks. My parents were concerned about my health and my mother was very unwell after the birth. For these reasons, my parents decided that they would not see my sister and asked the hospital to arrange a burial.

From the start, there appear to have been hints that the loss of my twin sister had affected me. I was a very unhappy baby, always crying and screaming. Often I would not be comforted or quietened by anything my parents did.

As a toddler I couldn't be left alone without becoming distressed. I am sure that this was a symptom of my bereavement. From what l have been told, I seem to have been particularly unable to cope with being left alone, or in a place where I couldn't see anyone else. I think I had an in-built fear of being abandoned again, as I had been in the womb. The consistent crying and colic I experienced as a baby are certainly recognised signs of trauma in utero.

I seemed to settle temporarily when my brother was born. I was just under three years old. Maybe it was to do with having a replacement for my sister. However, I have never had a close relationship with my brother.

The other 'complication' with regard to my sister, was my grandmother's belief in and practice of spiritualism. Although she never claimed to have contacted my sister at spiritualist meetings, she would often make a passing comment when we went to visit her that she had 'seen' my sister about the house.

I remember her talking about my sister in this way as long ago as when I was three or four years old. I don't think I was ever upset by it. In fact, I remember asking about what she looked like and being quite interested in what my grandmother had seen. However, I think that it could have been confusing for me. I do remember worrying about her reports of spiritualist meetings because I couldn't bring myself to believe that these things had actually happened and yet I couldn't believe my grandmother would lie to me either.

In a lot of ways I wish my Gran were still alive so that I could talk to her about it now. She died when I was thirteen. When I first started feeling that my sister was very important, I felt that my Gran could have done me a lot of harm, talking about seeing my sister as a ghost. However, there is a part of me now that is so grateful that she saw her as a real person and that she treasured her 'encounters' with her. I don't believe in spiritualism myself, but I'm sure that it was a great comfort to my grandmother, whether she actually saw her or only believed she did, and I don't begrudge her that. It seems strange though, that it still took me so many years to become conscious of how much losing my sister has affected me.

The effects have been deep and intense, at the very core of my soul. Perhaps the main result is that I have always felt very isolated and alone. I have had friends throughout my life, many of them close, but I've always felt an intense loneliness which nothing quenches. Although some of it is almost certainly due to other events in my childhood, I have always had a deep sense that it is much more than that. I have never understood why other people are happy with what seem to me to be superficial relationships. I've always felt that people never talk to each other at a level which really matters and that people are never 'themselves', which to me makes relationships pointless. I want relationships with other people which are empathic or even telepathic.

I find it very difficult when someone doesn't instinctively know what I am feeling. This results in some considerable frustration at times, but now that I know it is because I am wishing that I had a replacement for my sister, I can handle it much better, although it doesn't prevent me from wishing it was so. I have found that other people become anxious when their feelings begin to merge with another person's. That type of closeness often seems unbearably intrusive to people who were born as singletons, but to me it is how relationships should be, I suppose because that is how my relationship with my twin sister was. Some lines of T. S. Eliot's play, The Cocktail Party sum it up for me:

> It isn't that I want to be alone, but that everyone is alone, or so it seems to me. They make noises and they think they are talking to each other, they make faces and they think they understand each other, and I'm sure they don't. (1982 p.131)

As a child and even an adult, before I began to suspect the

effect of my sister's death on me I had feelings and images which I now believe were subconscious expressions of my feelings of loss. As a teenager, I would frequently draw a pale, thin girl with her arms outstretched as if reaching for something which wasn't there. I also had an incredibly powerful dream when I was about six or seven which is still very vivid. I dreamt that I was dead and I felt terrified. I was going to various adults, trying to get them to believe that I was dead and how frightened I was, but no one would listen to me. They all patted me on the head and told me to go away. Although part of the message seems to be the lack of understanding I felt, I think it must also say something about my dead twin.

More recently, when I was a day patient in hospital, I drew what is the most powerful image to me now, although incredibly, I didn't know why I was drawing it at the time. The picture is of a girl banging her fist against the mirror in frustration because there is no reflection of herself in it. This to me can be nothing other than an image reflecting my loss. There should have been a reflection – my identical twin sister - and she isn't there. The rediscovery of this drawing left me feeling shaken up and even now it makes me feel quite strange when look at it.

My time as a day patient was part of a long treatment for depression and anxiety from which I have suffered on and off since I was a child.

Because I wasn't finding the treatment I was given for depression at all helpful in the early stages, I began reading a great deal about psychology and, in particular, pre-birth experiences in the hope of finding some 'answers' for myself. Alice Miller's books have provided me with a lot of answers about my feelings - I think she is wonderful. It was her recommendation of the book *Making Sense of Suffering* by Konrad Stettbacher, (1990) that led me to read his views on

the effect of a person's birth on their emotional well-being.
I was scathingly sceptical at first and did not believe that
those sorts of feelings and memories could survive into
adulthood, but as I continued to read, feelings about my
sister began to come to the surface. I found myself thinking,
'If the births he is describing are classed as traumatic, what
was mine?' I shared the womb with my identical twin sister
(there can be no closer relationship). I was then lying next
to her dead body for several days without being able to
understand why she had stopped responding to me. She
then 'disappeared' (she was removed with forceps) and I
was dragged into the world the same way and isolated in a
special baby unit. Surely all of this was a deeply traumatic
experience, especially since a baby has no means of
comprehending what is happening except to have a severe
sense of loss and fear, of bewilderment and of feeling
suddenly very alone. A baby can not verbalise its feelings
and experiences, so those feelings can be elusive even when
the adult has learnt the vocabulary to interpret them verbally.
I have certainly found that this has compounded the problem
of coming to terms with being a lone twin, because the
feelings it produces are so difficult to express.

Once I had begun to consider the effects of being a lone
twin, I began to have very intense feelings of bereavement
and despair, but I was afraid to trust my feelings. I still
couldn't quite believe that my birth experiences could be
affecting me now. However, I was determined to find out
more about it so that I could discover whether it really is
possible to have feelings of grief years after an event and
whether it might possibly be contributing to my depression.

I contacted TAMBA (Twins and Multiple Births
Association.) I knew that this organisation is primarily for
parents of multiple birth children. However, they did put me
on to the bereavement group, who help parents who have lost

one or both twins at birth or in childhood. They in turn were
able to give me a few articles to read and put me in touch
with the Lone Twin Network.

I joined the Network in December 1992. It has been
helpful to read some of the articles they have been able to
send me. I have also been to two of their March meetings in
London. Both meetings were extremely helpful, even though
I did not find either meeting easy. I always find going to
strange places and meeting new people very difficult anyway,
and the meetings are always very emotional events.

Talking to other lone twins was far more than just
'interesting'. It brought all sorts of feelings even more to
the surface. It had really got too much by the afternoon, but
everybody knows what the feelings are like and everybody
supports each other.

I have already mentioned the effect on my perception
of relationships and my feelings of being intensely alone.
This seems to be quite common among the lone twins I
have met. There is certainly a general feeling of loss which
even having friends and relationships does not completely
address. However, it became obvious to me that I felt
this more intensely than the rest of the group I was with.
Someone asked me if I thought that being an identical twin
had made a difference. All the other people in my group
were non-identical twins. Of course, I had to answer that
I didn't know. But, although I know some of my feelings
may also be linked to other factors in my life, as I believe
is true of most people, I have come away from the meetings
with the impression that being an identical twin does seem
to have increased my feelings of isolation. In a way, I
suppose, it is logical. I teach quite a number of identical
and non-identical twins and I do sense quite a marked
difference in their relationships with each other. Identical
twins have a particularly intense form of communication.
It's almost verging on telepathy at times. For example, I

teach one pair of identical twins who would often argue because they each accused the other of copying their work, which was extremely similar, both in ideas and in the way they expressed them. But I knew that they had been sitting at opposite ends of the room for the whole lesson and it took a while for them to realise and accept that they had not knowingly copied each other. I know this is a very common experience for identical twins and this makes me believe that in the womb, too, there could be a particular closeness. That is not to say, of course, that non-identical twins can't be very close. I am also aware that not all twins, identical or non-identical, get on - I have seen this in other twins I have taught.

Connected with the feeling of isolation, there seemed to be a very common experience in lone twins of an inability to cope with loss, be it bereavement or simply the ending of a friendship, for whatever reason. This has always been a severe difficulty for me. I cannot cope with loss and change and I have never done so, even something as minor as a friend moving away. The only way that I can deal with it is to suppress the overwhelming feelings and then, of course, they fester for months afterwards and longer. It was once pointed out to me that I always seem to be abandoned and this *is* how it feels sometimes. I am sure these feelings are all the more intense because they echo my original abandonment pre-natally when my sister died.

However, paradoxically, I also feel that I abandoned my sister. This is an incredibly strong feeling at times and it makes me want to be able to hold her, protect her and comfort her. Although I know that a baby is in reality quite powerless over events, I feel as if, being the only one who knew her, I should have stayed with her, and that means that I desperately didn't want to be born. I think that I became very still and withdrawn in the womb after her death, as if trying to 'join' her, although I obviously wouldn't have understood that she was no longer responding to me because she was dead.

Difficulties in coping with loss and separation were too common at the Lone Twin meeting to be coincidence. I'm sure some people who are not lone twins also have difficulties with separation and loss, perhaps deriving from other factors in their personal history, but I'm convinced that the extent of the desperation which lone twins seem to feel regarding loss and the number of people at the meeting who expressed such intense feelings cannot be coincidence.

One person at the first meeting I attended, gave an account of how she always pushed herself relentlessly to give and give to others as if justifying her existence in some way. I certainly do find myself doing this and several others said they also identified with this feeling. As she pointed out, it's as if, subconsciously, we have to justify being alive because our twin did not survive and the only way of doing this is to endlessly give to others. I know that the reason I went into the teaching profession is because of the opportunities it gives for me to help the teenagers I teach. Of course, this is not a black and white situation. There is a right and proper part of me that genuinely wants to help the children I teach. But in the times when I have considered changing my profession, what has prevented me is that I see it as the only part of my life where I am making some attempt to 'atone' (I can think of no other word) for my existence, and most of the time, that still doesn't seem to be enough.

There seems to be a common feeling in lone twins that they are living for two, which in some ways must also be connected with the guilt of surviving, although it has a positive effect on some lone twins and gives them extra strength. Yet another aspect of lone twins which I noticed, was the large proportion of lone twins at the meetings who are in overtly caring professions such as nurses, teachers with a special interest in pastoral work and therapists.

It also seemed unlikely to me that there would normally be so large a percentage of people in a group who had either had or were in the throes of therapy for one reason or another. Not all lone twins end up in therapy, of course, and other factors play a part in leading people to therapy too.

Most of all, though, the similarity between lone twins I have met appears to be the depth of feeling and empathy for others which we as lone twins seem blessed (or cursed) with. There is quite a bit of disagreement about when babies begin to have a sense of me/not me, which is central to the development of their personalities, but I wonder whether twins develop this earlier than singletons, as they have another person (a 'not me' experience) to relate to from the start. If so, then I wonder if this can account in part for this highly developed empathy. This is a characteristic which I sensed incredibly strongly at the meeting. If there had been any doubt in my mind about there being such a thing as 'lone twinness', it was certainly dissipated by seeing this empathy in so many lone twins.

But it does also seem that the degree to which lone twins are adversely affected by their bereavement can be partly governed by the way it has been handled as they were growing up. Those whose parents have openly acknowledged and grieved for their dead baby, as well as loving the surviving one, seem to cope better with the loss and be less affected by it in adulthood. Some families have perfectly good reasons for not wishing to dwell on their dead baby, but instead concentrate on the living one and I am not criticising them for this. My parents did not dream that it would have such a lasting effect on me. As far as I know, there was nothing known about lone twins at the time I was born and no one could have been expected to know that it would affect me in the way it did. Although things have improved in more recent years, there are still far too many people who know nothing about the subject. Nevertheless, a lack of acceptance of a dead twin while the survivor grows up, does seem to compound the difficulties for those twins both in childhood and adulthood.

I have met a few lone twins who say that they haven't been affected by the loss of their sibling in any way and these people often seem to have families who have been very up-front about the death. Having said that, it makes me smile a little that they have all, without exception, gone on in the course of the conversation to talk about several aspects of their lives in which they have experienced feelings that are, in fact, very common in lone twins!

Since joining the Lone Twin Network, I have had the opportunity to read some studies of pre-natal experience in general, from which it is possible to gain more insight into how lone twins feel when they lose a brother or sister in the womb. It was such a relief to read the proof that memory of pre-natal and post-natal experiences can remain and be recalled well into adult life. The books reassured me that the original event did affect me as I grew up and that the more overt feelings that have now been reawakened in me with vehemence are real and have a concrete and accessible origin. I even have a strong sense that we lay close together, with her back curled against my stomach. When I get flashes of this image, it feels so real. I can 'feel' her skin and the warmth of her body and everything is quiet and so peaceful. It's very hard to describe the feeling adequately in words, but it is extremely vivid and moving. I often had the physical feeling that I had something missing the length of my body long before I had these memories and I have always felt very vulnerable there. I have modelled the two of us together as I feel we were in the womb in an attempt to capture the 'memory' in a more concrete way.

For a long time after I had joined the Network, I felt overwhelmed by the feelings that I was experiencing. I cannot describe them as anything other than severe grief, which I should have worked through a very long time ago. I have largely come to terms with losing her now, but I still think about her a great deal and the feelings of grief can be re-triggered. It feels so strange to be having these feelings so long after the event, but I now know why I feel them. I am a twin and nothing will take that away from me, but that also means that I can never be completely free of the effects of losing my sister.

Apart from meeting and talking with other lone twins, I have also been able to come to terms with my loss through actively seeking to create concrete symbols and memorials to her. It helped me a huge amount to draw a picture of us together as babies and to give her a name. I obviously am unable to have a photograph of her, so this was the next best thing. I knew that some people found comfort in finding or creating a grave for their lost twin. At first I couldn't begin to cope with the idea of doing this myself.

However, gradually I began to feel that I wanted to know where she was. I looked forward to possibly having a headstone put on the spot and taking a photograph of it. I had seen photos like this taken by two other lone twins at the March meeting. I wrote to the hospital where we were born and eventually the bereavement officer replied to me with the name of the cemetery where the hospital had buried her. I contacted the cemetery, hoping that they would be able to show me exactly where she was, but to my dismay, they wrote back to say that they could only show me a large grass area where the hospital buried babies and that they had no more detailed records. At first I couldn't accept this and all my plans of visiting her spot seemed completely meaningless. But eventually I decided go and another lone twin friend said she would meet me there, which I was incredibly grateful for, as I don't think I could have coped with it alone.

It felt very strange to be there and I couldn't stop crying, although I didn't really know what I was crying about and I felt very detached from it all. Funnily enough, I felt fine on my way home, but it all came out at four in the morning, when I woke up in a panic attack. My friend picked up a fir cone from the area where Sarah is buried and picked me some lavender and since then it has helped to have those things because they came from the place where she is.

A few weeks later I decided to buy one of the necklaces which come in two halves and to bury one half in the cemetery as near to where she is buried as I could. I would wear the other half so that I would always have a connection with her. I got permission to plant a small tree so that I could put the necklace underneath it. I did this a fortnight later and I also put a plaque there, which reads 'In Loving Memory of Sarah Lucy Goode, stillborn 4/12/63, Twin Sister of Bryony.' I felt that I needed to name her and let the world know that my little sister is buried there. I had been wearing both halves of the necklace since I had bought it and splitting up the two halves was a very emotional moment. I wear my part of the necklace all the time now and find it very comforting to look at and hold. It gives me a real sense of connection with Sarah and makes me feel complete somehow. The wording on the necklace, which is commonly used by friends who are to be apart for a while, seems incredibly appropriate for my situation. It reads, 'The Lord watch between me and thee while we are absent, one from another.' I carry a photograph of the tree and cemetery around with me and that also helps.

I told my parents that I had done all this. I wasn't sure how they would react, since they had chosen at the time of the original event not to commemorate her and I know they did this thinking they were doing the best thing. But they were pleased I had planted the tree and put up the plaque and, even though they don't want to visit the cemetery at the moment, they now have copies of the photographs that I took there.

Despite having taken all these steps to reclaim my sister, and there is no doubt that it has helped, I wanted her stillbirth certificate. In a way it seemed like the only official evidence that she existed, particularly since I have no photographs or possessions that belonged to her. I had not realised, however, that stillbirth certificates are different from death certificates. They are kept in Southport and, unlike death certificates for children who have lived even a few minutes, they will not issue stillbirth certificates to anyone other than the parents. They argue that, in the case of a stillbirth, the parents are the only ones to have been directly involved with the baby and that it was not anyone else's business. I was devastated. It felt like everyone was conspiring to keep every little part of her away from me. However, with perseverance and several letters later, the authorities were persuaded that in the case of a lone twin, who had shared a womb for several months with their brother or sister, the surviving twin had a right to have access to their twin's stillbirth certificate. I was the first lone twin to obtain this certificate and several others have since been permitted to have them also. It has made me feel that her existence has been truly acknowledged.

Although Sarah will always be a very large part of my life, and the effects of losing her will mean that I will always feel that a part of me is missing, I feel much more at peace now and able to accept her death. My necklace will remain my most treasured possession.

**Postscript:** Since writing this article, Sarah's memorial at the cemetery was lost. The cemetery manager agreed to replace it with a permanent stone plaque, engraved with the same wording as the original. Hopefully this one will withstand the test of time.

*Bryony Goode*

## NOTE FROM JOAN WOODWARD:

I appreciate this opportunity to confirm the views expressed in my book, *The Lone Twin: Understanding Twin Bereavement and Loss.* The research quoted in my book concerning memory starting in the foetus at around six months leads me to believe that the loss of a twin during the third trimester could for that reason have some significance for some twins. I still hold the view that it is probably the parental response to the loss that most influences the feelings of the surviving twin. I am convinced that how a mother feels about her baby during the pregnancy and birth does affect the child, whether these feelings are negative or positive. Significantly, nearly all the Lone Twins whose reaction was categorised by themselves as 'slight' thought that this was due to their mothers being relieved that there was only one baby. As a result these Lone Twins were considered to be 'very special'.

*Joan Woodward*
*Birmingham, 2006*

# THE WOMB/TOMB – A FEELING THROUGH TIME

No place, no time, just fear. No map to find a way.
I cannot see, I cannot feel, the void it all consumes.
There's no way out, there's no way in, a state within a mind.
A state to keep, a state to flee, a terror from all sides.
A burrowing deep inside the soul, a prison within, a prison
without, but never they shall meet.
A separation in the core that's buried deep, no access from
within, no access from without.
It keeps me safe, it keeps me born, it keeps me held in fear, a
ping-pong on a trip to hell with no way out of time.

How can I move without its grasp? How can I see within?
How can I find a way to be, a way away from me?
If I move out, if I move on, then I will cease to be, alone in
space without a space, a vacuum on the wind.
This is the way, the only way, without it I am done. I am not
here, I am not me, I am a never be.

It is a trust that's forged in blood, that this way I must be, for
if I'm not then I am not, I shatter wall to wall and drift off
into never land, some flotsam on the tide of time.
It's all there is, no way can go, no way I know, and yet I seek
a way, a way away from hurt and pain, a way away from
fear.

I must go through but how to start? What pattern can I forge?
What sequence in the past can forever lay my way and let the
devils rest?
A dark tomb looms from which I sense no exit will appear, a
journey unto my doom.

To feel my fate and yet to be, to feel the end of time and
from it start anew.
To plunge past the gates of my demise and emerge within
myself.
To cease to be in order to be me.
To chance the certainty of end, to be alone no more, to join
with me and there to start to be.

*© Richard Moore  July 2005*

~~~~~

*Richard Moore, Bsc (Hons) Psych, is a freelance editor and
poet living in the UK.  He and his wife share their home with
amazing  amounts of stuff and George the Dog.  Richard
believes he may be a wombtwin survivor.*

# PART TWO

## "VANISHING TWIN" PHENOMENON

# CHARLES E. BOKLAGE PH. D

## FREQUENCY AND SURVIVAL PROBABILITY OF NATURAL TWIN CONCEPTIONS

*Twin pregnancy ends with a single birth more then with twins; the concept of the 'vanishing twin syndrome' (or phenomenon) has attracted considerable attention over the past several years. In reality, however, losing one or both offspring from a twin pregnancy is too common to be called phenomenal, and occurs for too many different reasons to qualify as a syndrome.*

~~~~~

Charles Boklage is a professor in the Department of Pediatrics in the Brody School of Medicine and adjunct professor of biology at East Carolina University. He has studied the development and genetic make-up of twins for the past 20 years. He is a prolific writer on matters related to twinning.

*(Extracts from book chapter reproduced with permission of the publisher.)*

*Keith, L.G., Papiernik, E., Keith, D.M. and Luke, B. (eds) (1995) Multiple Pregnancy: Epidemiology, Gestation and Perinatal Outcome. New York: Parthenon. Chapter 4, pp. 41-2, 49*

# 8

# FREQUENCY AND SURVIVAL PROBABILITY OF NATURAL TWIN CONCEPTIONS

*Charles E. Boklage*

## Introduction

Most human pregnancies never reach term, as they fail before clinical recognition. The same is true for twin pregnancies. Optimised projections using available data indicate term survival of no more than one in four natural conceptions, and no more than one in 50 natural twin pairs. These projections also indicate that one pregnancy in eight begins as twins, and that, for every live born twin pair, 10-12 twin pregnancies result in single births. Using these estimates, 12-15% of all live births are products of twin embryogenesis. Twin pregnancy ends with a single birth more often than with twins; the concept of the 'vanishing twin syndrome' (or phenomenon) has attracted considerable attention over the past several years.[1, 2, 3] In reality, however, losing one or both offspring from a twin pregnancy is too common to be called phenomenal and occurs for too many different reasons to qualify as a syndrome. The concept found its present name in 1980, at the Third International Congress on Twin Studies in Jerusalem. Elizabeth Noble, who went on to explore the psychology of surviving the early loss of a twin [4] asked the question that provoked the discussion. One or both of the Keith twins interjected the term 'vanishing twins.' Their later paper with Landy [2] assaying the scope of the problem and labelling the event for the literature, followed from that discussion. The actual quantitation of losses from twin pregnancies remains, however a relatively small part of a more general problem, for which we recently published a plausible statistical approach.[5]

The causes, frequency and timing of prenatal losses are of interest at several levels, none of which is unique to twins. Despite this, understanding these processes can help clarify the epidemiology and developmental biology of twinning and numerous anomalies of human reproduction associated with twinning either in individuals or in families. If, for example, the risk of prenatal death for the individual member of a multiple pregnancy were identical to that for a single pregnancy, multiple pregnancies appear to suffer greater losses for the simple reason that more lives are at risk. Although this likelihood must be considered in any proper analysis, considerable data indicate that multiple pregnancies are in fact at greater risk from a variety of sources.[3] The nature and extent of the excess for each or both twins(s) are difficult to define precisely, but remain worthy of our best efforts at understanding.[5, 7-9]

**Looking forward**

The increasing use of transvaginal ultrasonography should provide earlier detection of multiple pregnancy as well as better viability prognosis.[21] Its use, combined with serial assay of HCG [22-24], should make it possible to detect twin pregnancies at least nearly as early as single pregnancies. Application of these techniques in a sample of sufficient size should provide much more straightforward and more accurate answers to all of these present questions.

There is little room to doubt that the question of vanishing twins and sole survivors of twin gestation represents issues or broad and fundamental importance. The numbers estimated here for the frequency of twinning at conception and the prevalence of sole survivors of twin gestations are little short of astonishing at first consideration, and they are conservative, perhaps even minimum, estimates. To expect significant improvement in these estimates will require obstetricians in the field to collect sound data using early non-invasive means with careful documentation, so that we may calculate these rates with improved confidence.

# References

## Introduction

1. Alexander, T.P. (1987). *Make Room for Twins*. (New York: Bantam Books)

2. Landy, H.J., Keith,L.G. and Keith, D. (1982). The Vanishing Twin. *Acta Genet. Med. Gemellol.*, 31,179

3. MacGillivray, I., Campbell, D.M. and Thompson. B. (1988) *Twinning and Twins*. ( New York: John Wiley & Sons)

4. Noble, E. (1991) *Having Twins* 2nd edition (Boston: Houghton Mifflin)

5. Boklage, C.E. (1990). Survival probability of human conceptions from fertilization to term. *Internation J. Fertil.*, 35, 75

6. Boklage C.E. (1987) Twinning, non righthandedness, and fusion malformations . Evidence for heritable causal elements held in common. *Am. J. Med Genet.* 28,67

7. Boklage C.E. (1987) Race zygosity and mortality between twins: interaction of myth and method. *Acta. Genet. Med. Gemellol.* 36 275

8. Boklage, C.E. (1985) Interactions between opposite-sex dizygotic fetuses and the assumptions of Weinberg difference method epidemiology. *Am. J. Hum. Genet.* 37, 591

9. Bryan E.M. (1986) The intrauterine hazards of twins *Arch.Dis.Child.* 61, 1044

## Looking forward

21. Pampiglione J.S. and Mason, B.A. (1988) Fetal viabiity in multiple pregnancy. *Lancet* 2, 554

22. Thiery, M., Dhont, M. and Vandekerckhove, D. (1977) Serum HCG and HPL in twin pregnancies. *Acta Obstet.Gynecol. Scand.,* 56, 495

23. Bernaschek, G., Rudelstorfer, R. and Csaicsich,P. (1988) Vaginal sonography versus serum human chorionic gonadotrophon in early detection of pregnancy *Am. J. Obstet. Gynecol.* 158, 608

24. Kelly, M.P., Molo, M.W., Maclin,V.M. et al. (1991) Human chorionic gonadotrophin rise in normal and vanishing twin pregnancies. *Fertil. Steril.,* 56, 221

# LIFE IN DEATH

I'm here and yet it is not there for me
I touch and yet I cannot feel
I live though I am not alive
I speak
And merely hear the shadow of myself
Echoing

And if I see a green around me
Deep soft cushioned
And dark and striking green
I know it's reaching out for me
It beckons me to be there in its midst
I want to be.  I would be
But no
I cannot be
For I'm surrounded
Shut up
Skin tight
In life in death

*Nick Owen*

~~~~~

*This is the Dead Twin aspect of the self, the world is just
beyond my reach, just beyond my reality.  It was still many
years before I realised I had lost a twin in the womb.*

© *Nick Owen 1970*

# DR KERRON HARVEY

## WHAT VANISHING TWINS MAY BE TELLING US

*For years, cerebral palsy was attributed to injury during
a difficult birth, but research has shown that this is seldom
the case. Studies conducted by Dr Peter Pharoah, a
University of Liverpool scientist, now suggest that
the damage is inflicted early in pregnancy – and it may
be linked to a co-twin 'vanishing' during the first trimester.
If further research supports this hypothesis, it may be
possible one day to reduce surviving twins' risk of
suffering from cerebral palsy.*

~~~~~

Dr Kerron Harvey is contributing editor of *Research
Intelligence,* a quarterly newsletter, published by
The University of Liverpool.

Dr Peter Pharoah is an Emeritus Professor at The Universiy
of Liverpool, specialising in maternal and child health issues
and perinatal epidemiology.

*Complete article (minus original illustrations) previously published in
Research Intelligence, Issue 17, August 2003
(see http://www.liv.ac.uk/researchintelligence/issue17/vanishingtwins.html)*

# 9

## WHAT VANISHING TWINS MAY BE TELLING US

*Dr Kerron Harvey*

Most of us have a broad understanding of the evolutionary theory based on survival of the fittest – i.e. the best adapted – organisms. We know that 'natural selection' has been at work for millions of years, and that it has shaped the evolution of modern humans.

We may prefer not to think about it, but it is still at work today – impacting on our own lives. It is the driving force behind a fascinating phenomenon known as 'vanishing twins'. These are twins who appear on early ultrasound scans, only to disappear before the follow-on scan a couple of months later. It's a common phenomenon in pregnancies following fertility treatment – but it also happens in naturally occurring pregnancies. Until recently, we knew very little about vanishing twins. Now, thanks to painstaking research by Liverpool University scientists, we're gaining insights into the numbers involved, the likely causes – and the implications for surviving co-twins.

### Evidence from different sources

Midwives have known for years that occasionally a tiny, fully-formed fetus is attached to the placenta at birth, as well as the son or daughter the parents expected. It is usually dry and papery, is known as a 'fetus papyraceus', and is all that remains of a dead twin. Today, ultrasound technology can identify twins in the first trimester of pregnancy. However, hospitals don't usually tell mothers at this stage, and they may not even record the twins' existence; vanishing twins are sufficiently common that hospitals prefer to avoid triggering feelings of loss, grief or guilt in mothers whose scans at 20 weeks reveal only singletons. And yet, if Emeritus Professor Peter Pharoah is right, this information could be vital to the wellbeing of both twins.

## Link to cerebral palsy

Peter Pharoah is a medic, an epidemiologist and a member of Liverpool University's Department of Public Health. In the mid-1990s, he was studying the fates of twin pairs where one twin was known to have died during pregnancy. He discovered that the prevalence of cerebral palsy in the surviving twins was over fifty times higher than normal.

Historically, the condition was thought to result from injury during a difficult birth, but research has shown that this is seldom the case. In the light of his findings, Peter Pharoah and his colleague, Professor Richard Cooke, proposed that cerebral palsy is largely attributable to the death of a co-twin – by stillbirth or by vanishing.

"Essentially, we were suggesting that cerebral palsy in apparently singleton babies is most likely to be due to a former twin who vanished early in the pregnancy", Peter Pharoah explains.

Identical twins come from a single fertilized egg which splits into two embryos. If the egg divides very early – up to, say, three days following fertilization, each twin could have its own placenta, chorion and amniotic sac. If they split any later than this, they will share their placenta; they could share their chorion; and they could even share the amniotic sac; in all these cases, they will invariably share their blood supply.

Peter Pharoah believes that when this happens, blood can sometimes shunt to and fro between the twins, and this can damage one or both of them. If this happens very early in the development of the fetus, it may affect organs like the heart, kidney or intestines; the damage may even kill one twin. Variation in the blood supply may also affect the brain, and its precise timing may influence the type of brain impairment suffered.

## Testing the hypothesis

Peter Pharoah set out to test his hypothesis regarding the cause of cerebral palsy. Initially, he relied on secondary data, but this proved to be problematical. "If a vanishing twin is expelled from the womb before 24 weeks, there's no legal requirement to record the birth or the death", he explains. "If it's expelled after 24 weeks, the birth certificate may record its sex as 'indeterminate' – or the parents may be allowed to record the sex of their choice, which skews the data. The death certificate may simply say 'congenital abnormality', without any indication what form this took."

Nonetheless, this approach has enabled Peter Pharoah to show that the risk of live twins being born with cerebral palsy is five times higher than it is for live singletons. Where co-twins are known to have died in the womb, the prevalence of cerebral palsy in the surviving twin is ~82 per 1000, compared to an overall prevalence of ~2 per 1000 live births.

## Numbers of vanishing twins

Information on vanishing twins and the fate of their co-twins can be extracted from mothers' pregnancy and children's own health records, but this doesn't necessarily provide the comprehensive information Peter Pharoah requires.

"We need to know whether twins were identical or non-identical, and whether identical twins shared a chorion", he explains, "but this is not always recorded."

To overcome this problem, Peter Pharoah is collaborating with clinicians at Liverpool Women's Hospital. They are recording the data he needs on twin pregnancies revealed by ultrasound scans at 11-12 weeks, and checking whether both twins are still visible on ultrasound scans made 20 weeks into the pregnancy. Peter Pharoah's analysis of the first year's data suggests that twins occur at a rate of 120 per 1000 pregnancies in the UK.

"Data from the Office of National Statistics show that only 80 pairs of twins are delivered per 1000 live births in the UK", he says. "That's roughly a third fewer than there probably were at the start of the pregnancy. Stillbirths account for some of this discrepancy, but we're still left with a twin vanishing in 30 per 1000 pregnancies. A minority are mono-chorionic – possibly enough to explain the prevalence of cerebral palsy. Vanishing twins may also explain other neurological disability and birth defects – like absent kidneys, heart malformations and gut blockages.

Peter Pharoah would like to extend his research to encompass these conditions. He would also like to identify mothers carrying twins at the earliest possible opportunity – around, say, 6-8 weeks. "There's evidence to suggest that some mono-chorionic twins are vanishing before 11-12 weeks, when the first ultrasound scans are taken", he explains. "To test my hypothesis, we would need to take account of this."

If further research supports his hypothesis, it may be possible one day to prevent either twin from suffering the damaging – and possibly fatal – consequences of sharing a chorion.

# IN THE VALLEY

In the valley of the shadow of death
I walk into the light of my Beloved
Into my eternal heartbreak of longing
I am led by the shadows of moonlight
And silver-green melodies of singing whispers,
An absolving memory,
I fall into Your Heart,
I am pierced once again,
I find Your door
Stumble in,
Darkly,
You are not home,
My Soul is absent,
It is here my breath remains.


*Ana Ruiz*


~~~~~


*I know relatively little about womb twins, but I do know
about a sense of profound loss, a sense of missingness, of
trying to find something to fill in the blanks of this emptiness.
It has been my journey of a lifetime, coming to terms with my
absolute aloneness.*


© *Anna Ruiz 2005*

## CORTNEY DAVIS MA, RNC, APRN

## WHERE DID IT GO?

*While I understand much of the biology of the vanishing
twin phenomenon, it's a mystery of nature that
intrigues me. I wonder how many of us might
have once been two, not one.*

~~~~~

Cortney Davis is a nurse practitioner working in women's
health. She is a prolific writer and has published several
books and articles about issues of medical care, including
an award-winning book entitled *I Knew a Woman: the
Experience of the Female Body,* which is a memoir of her
work as a nurse practitioner, and three books of poetry. She
has given readings and writing seminars all over the USA an
has been interviewed on several radio and TV channels.

*Article previously published in
Discover Magazine, Vol. 23, No. 10, October 2002
Reproduced with the permission of the author.*

# 10

## WHERE DID IT GO?

*Cortney Davis*

On the ultrasound screen, I could see 11-week-old twins—two shadows, like reflected commas, suspended in the patient's uterus. One embryo moved its arm. The other, slightly smaller, squirmed and floated head up. When I pointed them out, Linda was both shocked and overjoyed. "I can't believe it!" she said. "I'm going to have twins!"

She propped herself on her elbows to see, the table paper crinkling beneath her. Outside the exam room door, the waiting room was filled with other pregnant women waiting for their exams. But here was an event. Twins.

In the women's center where I work as a nurse practitioner, we see twin gestations several times a year. We don't often see identical twins, but the occurrence of fraternal twins, resulting from the fertilization of two eggs by two different sperm, is more common and varies according to race, genetic factors, maternal age, and the use of fertility drugs. Once, we had a real surprise—fraternal twins fathered by two different men. In that case, the patient's two eggs had been fertilized by different partners, a rare occurrence that results when separate acts of intercourse take place within a brief period of time.

Linda's twins appeared to be fraternal—we could see that the embryos were encased in separate membranes—and her predisposition to twins was probably age-related: Linda was 39. Although it seems logical that twins would occur less frequently as women age, the opposite is true. The more pregnancies a woman has carried and the older she is, the more likely she is to conceive twins. An increase in one of the reproductive hormones that helps eggs mature, FSH, is probably responsible for the increased chance of bearing twins.

I told Linda we would schedule another ultrasound at 18 weeks and that during the pregnancy we'd monitor the growth of the babies with monthly ultrasounds. She understood that a twin pregnancy was more vulnerable than a singleton. Intrauterine fetal demise, premature delivery, and discordant growth of the twins were all distinct possibilities. In addition, because of Linda's age, her pregnancy was at a higher risk for genetic abnormalities. She was nonetheless encouraged by the ultrasound; she carried the sonogram picture of her twins in her wallet and showed it to everyone.

When she was 13 weeks pregnant, Linda returned to the clinic for a routine check. The resident who examined her at that time located two strong fetal heartbeats. Two weeks later, when Linda was 15 weeks pregnant, I picked up her chart, happy to have the chance to see her again. She was animated, and we chatted about the Internet exploration she'd been doing. She had started e-mailing other women with twins, gone window-shopping for strollers, and subscribed to a magazine for families with twins. Loving the idea of having twins, she'd already begun thinking in pairs — a double stroller, two cribs, two bikes, and, eventually, two college educations.

First, I felt Linda's enlarged belly. Then, after slathering her abdomen with lubricant, I listened for two distinct fetal heart tones. I found one twin's heartbeat right away. It was strong and steady at 140 beats per minute, exactly in the normal range of 120 to 160; fetuses, like other small creatures, have rapid heart rates. Linda and I smiled.

The sound was like the gallop of a faraway pony or the wing beats of a hummingbird. Normally, it would have taken me only a moment or two to locate the other twin's heartbeat, but the minutes dragged on. No matter how intently I listened or how carefully I maneuvered the Doppler stethoscope over Linda's belly, I could find only one fetal heartbeat.

Linda asked, "What's the matter?"

My own heart was pounding as I tried to reassure her: "It's possible that I'm just not able to track down the second fetus. They move around pretty quickly."

I didn't remind her that the miscarriage rate is high in twin pregnancies, so much so that women often lose one twin before they even know they are expecting. I didn't say that in one study, twin pregnancies were identified in 30 women but only 14 resulted in the birth of two infants. Or that I'd read that when twins were seen on women's early ultrasounds, less than 50 percent of those women went on to deliver two babies.

Linda and I moved to the ultrasound room. When we looked at the screen, we could see that one twin was viable, moving and rolling, but the other was shrunken and still. I hugged Linda as she wept.

I assured her that this was not the result of anything she had done, nor was this necessarily a harbinger of disaster for the other fetus. I told her we would do what we usually do: wait. In the back room, the residents and I no longer spoke of Linda's two fetuses but referred to the one that had silently succumbed as the "conceptus" or the "demise."

The next ultrasound showed that the viable fetus was thriving. This one was female, her features identifiable and her sex clearly visible. The discrepancy was marked: in one sac, a baby girl; in the other sac, the conceptus, like a dark half-moon. I gave Linda all the details I could: how many weeks the other fetus had lived, how its minuscule body might eventually become compressed into the membranes, or how it might be delivered alongside her daughter.

Four weeks later, I expected to see an even more discordant picture as Linda's baby girl continued to grow, dwarfing the conceptus. But the ultrasound revealed only the healthy child. The dead fetus, the failed twin, the forever-unknowable child, had vanished, leaving behind, like a cast-off jacket, its empty sac. "Where did it go?" Linda asked, feeling her loss anew.

While the very early miscarriage or arrested growth of one developing ovum is common, what happened to Linda—the total disappearance of a twin later in pregnancy—is unusual. I gave her the simplistic explanation given in medical texts: "It was reabsorbed. Your body has absorbed the tissue." Weeks later, a final ultrasound showed that the sac was gone as well.

When Linda gave birth to her daughter at 38 weeks, there was no evidence of any kind that another embryo had ever existed—not a thickening in the placenta nor a small fetus hanging by a slender cord from the healthy twin's placenta. If Linda had not kept that early sonogram picture, there would be no way to prove that the vanished twin had ever been conceived.

As bewildered as if she'd accidentally misplaced some precious object, Linda believed that her body had reclaimed the dead fetus in order to keep it forever.

Six weeks after the delivery, she came into the clinic for her postpartum checkup. Her daughter, Carolina, was strong and healthy. Would Linda, I wondered, ever tell this child that once in a briny past she had had a sibling? Would this remaining child sometimes sense, as Linda surely must, the presence of the vanished twin?

While I understand much of the biology of the vanishing twin phenomenon, it's a mystery of nature that intrigues me. I wonder how many of us might have once been two, not one.

# PART THREE

## DO WE REMEMBER
## THE WOMB?

# ALTHEA HAYTON

## MARTHA : A CASE STUDY

*This case study illustrates how a simple conversation by
email can be very helpful for wombtwin survivors. "Martha"
began with a simple question: was overweight connected to
being a wombtwin survivor? I was glad to try and answer
this question, because it was something I had wondered
about too. Although the internet is a very public space,
it has the advantage of being anonymous. By this means
Martha was able to reveal some of her secret thoughts
and share them with me. Over the space of a year or two,
she gradually revealed - to both of us - how some vague
impressions of her life in the womb were driving her choices
and decisions in born life .*

~~~~~

Martha lives in Washington state, USA

*An original, previously unpublished article, compiled from a series
of emails, which were exchanged in the process of carrying out the
"Wombtwin work" with a woman who offered to take part in my research.*

*www.wombtwin.com*

# 11

## MARTHA: A CASE STUDY

*Althea Hayton*

*Martha came to me because of her problems with overweight.*

I hear talk about eating disorders like anorexia and bulimia being connected with vanished twin syndrome, but I don't hear of obesity. I don't seem to be able to "not eat" when I am alone. It's as though I am trying to find company and comfort in food and then when I overeat, there is the self-loathing that I'm so used to. Are you doing research in this area? I'd really love to participate.

*It sounded like a great deal of work had been done, but there was still a certain Something Else that needed to be aired and talked through.*

I had a twin brother who died around 4 months into the pregnancy, my mother has passed away and so I cannot ask her for any information about the pregnancy. I do know that she was hospitalised with the polio virus at the time of my birth and so I was placed in isolation for a time in the hospital as a new-born. I don't know how long, exactly. I was then cared for by relatives for a few months (possibly close to a year) until my mother could come home from the hospital and care for me. I always thought my "issues" were from the lack of bonding due to the isolation after birth.

My chiropractor helped me discover my brother and the emotional release that came as a result even before she explained to me what a "vanished twin" was... Well, it was an amazing experience. Learning about my twin made me feel that I had finally found the answer to my being whole and complete. I felt that knowing about him was the answer to the searching I had been doing all my life and I knew that I would someday be reunited with him.

I was sure that with this knowledge I would now be able proceed through the rest of my life and no longer feel the despair and longing for a release from the pain of being alone, but I still find myself mourning him, mourning my other failed relationships and feeling alone - even in a group of people who I would call friends, if I felt I really had friends.

This is the first time I've told a total stranger about myself and I thank you for the opening to do so. My twin has been with me a lot lately. I find that I've been drawn to look for things to represent my "twin-ness" in my life. Greeting cards with two indian figures represented, rubber stamps that show two hands reaching for each other, drawing two similar objects. Somehow this search both fills and unsettles me, but maybe it will help me on my way to being whole and complete without him. I find I want to talk about him a lot and on the odd occasion that I do, people seem to get confused and uncomfortable in the conversation.

I've been kind of "observing" my food patterns, self-promises, inability to fulfill those promises. I've been looking back at the emotional connection I've had with food throughout my life - but I've been avoiding doing any writing about what's in my head. It feels like some sort of "fear" of what will truly show up when it's put into print. I really want to move forward in my life. I feel like I'm caught in a spiral. I get strong and begin to move powerfully forward and then I get stopped by feelings of being incomplete and therefore unworthy of having the things in my life that I want. For example: I'm trying to start a business and I take two or three steps forward; I am inspired and people are enrolled in my project and then I just stop taking action that will move me forward. I fall back a step or two and find myself drifting and feeling incomplete. Before long nothing is happening to move my business forward and all forward momentum of business building is gone...

*I asked her to complete a simple diagnostic form and an additional ten questions, which revealed more.*

It was really strange, I felt the questions on the list were talking specifically about me. Pain, shame and intimacy: these are the areas that I use food to fill in my feelings of loss. Pain is a constant, which I feed. Then I feel Shame about overeating and being fat. Then the Shame keeps me away from Intimacy because of fear of more Pain... and so the cycle continues. This cycle is repeated on so many levels of my life. Not only food, friends, family, but in business and in achieving my life goals.

I've been thin before and I know that it still cycles - just not feeling as heavy a measure of shame when I was "looking good." I am concerned that my emotional roller-coaster is hampering my ability to stay on a healthy eating and exercise plan. I always say that if I had a "buddy" to do it with, I could succeed, but then the buddies don't work out for one reason or another. I think I'm looking for my twin to help me lose weight! I also feel that my weight is a shield that I have created to hide behind so that I will look the part of a flawed person and that I won't have to be the powerful, intelligent woman that I know myself capable of being.

I also have the relationship cycles of intense connection and then they dwindle away into nothing and then failure. I have learned in the last year or so that I sabotage my relationships, but have not yet learned how to get out of the negative behaviour cycles when I feel them start.

I have a serious emotional reaction to the death of a loved one. It gets worse every time. Very traumatic, but I also have issues about feeling that death (in relationship to myself) would be a release from the pain I feel at having survived. I have shame around body image, shame around food consumption, shame around making promises to myself and not being able to fulfill them. Outside of myself, however, I follow through on my promises to others and will practically hurt myself to be sure it happens. (Of course, if my promise to others doesn't happen, then it's my fault and there is shame again.)

I have abandonment issues, always searching for something or someone, but I do know I was and am loved. Larger than that, is that I have a sense of not belonging even when I know that I really am part of a group. I don't trust people either. So there is always that lack of trust as a barrier to intimacy. My feeling is that I will get hurt by my friend/ lover or the person that I love will go away.

*She mentioned her wombtwin by name, and in a curiously indifferent way: she wrote his name in quotation marks.*

You're right about the quotation marks around Matthew's name when I responded to the survey. I hadn't thought much about it. I don't think he is a fairy tale. He lives in my heart as truth - I do notice that when I speak of him, however, I say that I "believe myself to be" a wombtwin survivor. I see that I don't actually acknowledge that it is true, just something I believe to be true.

I guess that way of speaking is to protect myself in some way. I've had beliefs of other things that I thought were true and then found that my beliefs changed as I got more facts. I don't think this is the case here, but it's more of a habit pattern of qualifying my answers instead of asserting what I know as truth. The quotation marks could have been reflective of that speech pattern/habit, but I wonder if I may feel that I've only made him up.

I want to be free from whatever is holding me back in my life. So, I hereby choose to acknowledge my brother,

Matthew, as real, loved and missed. He is real in my heart.
I know he is not physically here in my present life, but very
much present in my thoughts. I talk to him occasionally
when I'm driving or home alone.

*Later, she mentioned her twin brother again and gave him*
*the name of "Michael". I asked her about that.*

Wow! I don't know where "Michael" came from, but it
was so smooth I didn't notice. I'm going to try-on Michael
and see if that's his real name. I felt good about Matthew
at the time, but I was "looking" for a name, because I felt I
should... Michael just came out on its own. I'm also open
to discover whether there was possibly that more than one
brother was lost.

Intellectually, I know that I'm whole and complete,
perfect as I am and the only one holding me back is me.
But sometimes it is a hard place to live with ghostlike
feelings (voices?) of guilt, loss, searching and similar
emotions that seem to have no basis in fact or experience to
cause them to be so powerful. It's not that I've had a bad or
hard life - it's really been quite a good life when compared
to the struggles of many, many others. I've never been
homeless. I've never been without food or love. I did have
discipline as a child, but not abusively.

The bottom line is that I feel as though I've lived a full
life. There have been some extreme highs and lows, but I've
known myself to be a survivor since the death of my older
brother in 1967. I wonder if that's something I've really
known all my life - now that I know about my twin.

I went through a pretty deep depression a couple
of years before the end of my marriage (about the third
or fourth time in my adult life that I remember) - I got
counselling for it this time and also started some Landmark
Education personal growth classes. It's those classes
that I say have helped me regain my personal power. My

Landmark classes have helped me see that I've carried this "I'm not good enough" through my life for as long as I can remember. It was simply as how I viewed myself. Some of my actions were also about looking to be loved. It's almost as if I were asking (without words) throughout my life "Do you love me?" and when the answer wasn't enough to convince me that they did, it was because "I'm not good enough" or "not worthy" to be loved and taken care of.

I find that I'm now looking toward the future, my business growth, my being able to again have a home of my own and to, once again, save for the future. It's empowering, exciting, fun, scary in a challenging sort of way, but I still have a little voice in my head that says I just want to be treasured and taken care of. A very small child sort of voice. It's getting smaller and quieter as my personal power has grown, but it's still where a part of me wants to go...

Not much is happening with my weight yet. I was struggling with it and making myself "wrong" for not being able to get it under control and then a friend who has been a hypnotherapist for 30 years approached me about doing some desk-top publishing for him. We've worked out a trade for services and he is helping to free my personal power to make better food choices and has helped me sleep better. I feel a lot better physically and know that I am making slow progress. I feel better, I'm more inclined to feel happy than inadequate these days. I'm sure the weight will begin to fall away as I continue to make better food and exercise choices.

I hold most of my weight on my stomach, like a blanket over my belly. I sort of look like I'm pregnant, but at 53, it's obvious that it's just fat. It's heavy when turning over at night. It gets in my way when I want to bend over. It doesn't really feel like part of me, just something that gets in the way. By now, the fat is moving to the rest of me too (face, thighs, etc.) but for a long time, everything else still looked reasonably thin and in decent physical condition.

It's only been in the last few years that I'm beginning to notice arms, legs, face carrying the fat too. I used to be able to camouflage my fat pretty well - not possible now. I had a dream last night that I was removing it like a coat. I just slipped it off and stepped out of it. A great dream!

## Post script

*After a break of many months I made contact with Martha again to ask her if I may use her story in this book.*

The conversation we had not long ago really added to my knowledge of what is or might be true to my situation, starting with the Matthew/Michael naming of my twin(s) and forward through the latest questionnaire that you sent out. I related to a lot of what you wrote about us. I think you are correct that I am the fraternal twin survivor of identical twins who vanished early in the pregnancy.

I am still single and not in a romantic relationship. My divorce was two years ago and I am creating a circle of friends that I enjoy and trust. I wouldn't be surprised to have a romantic relationship in the future, but don't feel in a hurry to find it. I'm enjoying working on finding balance in my life - socially, financially and professionally right now. I'm enjoying my friends and am happy with that at this time. Most of them are involved in the Landmark Education personal growth work that I've been participating in for the last 3 years or so - that has enabled me to live in what's possible instead of the sadness of what felt was missing in my life. Inside of this group of friends and the self-empowerment education that I've been getting, it's been interesting to watch my trust of people, particularly men, grow little by little.

I have my own place now, quiet and peaceful. A refuge from the hubbub of life. I find that having a place to go to rest and recover from the stress of daily life is a requirement for me to continue to move forward. If I don't have my own "space" I never feel fully recharged. I need to have a certain amount of alone time to recharge. Being in a group of people is always tiring for me. I know people who are "fed" by being in a group, I'm "fed" by being alone in my own space.

As far as my weight loss issue, I've worked closely with my Naturopathic doctor and discovered that my eating habits were not good for my blood sugar levels and so I've been having quite good success with a low sugar diet. I feel great. I'm below 250 pounds for the first time in 3 years and plan to be a hundred pounds lighter before I'm finished. I'm no longer hiding behind my blanket of belly fat.

I know that I "belong" in my life and that I can love and be loved by my family and friends safely. The feeling of "not having done enough" or "not being good enough" is still there now and then, but I now recognize it and can set it aside and move powerfully forward with what I've learned about myself and others. I thank you, my cousin and Landmark Education for that. I have tools to use to move forward and I'm glad to be alive.

## Recent update

*Some time later I received another update. Depression had returned because it was time to grieve. For wombtwin survivors, there are mood swings and healing is a long road.*

The discovery of my twin status was like opening a door and finding the reason and/or understanding for a lot of my behaviors and emotions over the years. It was like turning on the light. What I didn't know was that I still had a lot of work to do with this newly found knowledge. I couldn't just close the door and be "cured" and move on with this magic information in my pocket.

Since we last wrote, I've spiraled into another cycle of

severe depression. What has come up for me is the need to grieve for the lost twins - which I'm doing. It feels so right to just "be with" them and mourn their passing. No survivor guilt at the moment, just pure grief for them not being here. I am honoring them in my heart and crying when the need arises.

I feel this is something that was missing in my healing process before. I thought I was doing them honor, but I think I was doing what I "thought I should do" and not letting it all really get into my heart. I'm much more aware of my having created a continuation of alone-ness in my life and am looking for a way to connect with people to create a community to interact with regularly so that I can learn to be part of a group and not keep myself separated as I have done in the past.

I thank you for the validation I've felt by being part of your study of vanishing twins/wombtwin survivors.

*Over the years, it has been finding a supportive and helpful group that has helped Martha the most. After all, if she is indeed a triplet survivor, and lived in a little group for the first four months of her life, then recreating that group will help to heal that deep sense of loss and isolation.*

# DAVID CHAMBERLAIN PH.D

## BABIES ARE CONSCIOUS

*Newborn babies have been trying for centuries to convince us they are like the rest of us, sensing, feeling, thinking human beings. Struggling against thousands of years of ignorant supposition that newborns are partly human, sub-human, or not-yet human, the vast majority of babies arrive in hospitals today, greeted by medical specialists who still doubt that they can actually see, feel pain, have real emotions, learn, remember, or understand anything that happens to them.*

~~~~~

David Chamberlain is one of the founders of the Association for Prenatal and Perinatal Psychology and Health (APPPAH) and is editor of the website birthpsychology.com that attracts a thousand visitors daily from 100 countries. He lectures internationally, conducts workshops on prenatal psychology, and is an expert in hypnotherapy, trauma resolution and brief intensive therapy. His popular book, *The Mind of Your Newborn Baby*, is now in its 3rd edition (1998) in twelve languages.

*This paper was prepared in 1996 and published online in Jane English, Cesarean Voices (www.eheart.com/cesarean/babies.html) It was lightly revised in 2003 for publication in The Italian Journal of Psychology and Prenatal Education. Reproduced with permission of the author.*

# 12

## BABIES ARE CONSCIOUS

*David Chamberlain Ph.D*

Newborn babies have been trying for centuries to convince us they are like the rest of us sensing, feeling, thinking human beings. Struggling against thousands of years of ignorant supposition that newborns are partly human, sub-human, or not-yet human, the vast majority of babies arrive in hospitals today greeted by medical specialists who are still skeptical as to whether they can actually see, feel pain, learn, and remember what is done to them. Physicians, immersed in protocol, employ painful procedures, confident that no permanent impression, certainly no lasting damage will result from the manner in which babies are brought into this world.

The way medical doctors see infants (a view which may not be shared by women, midwives or doulas) has taken on increasing importance in countries where 95% are born in a hospital and perhaps 30% or more are delivered surgically. While this radical change was occurring in the Western world over the last half century, the psychological aspects of birth were not generally considered. In fact, for most of the 20th century, medical beliefs about the infant nervous system were accepted automatically in psychology. However, in the last three decades, psychology has invested heavily in infant studies and uncovered many previously hidden talents of both the fetus and the newborn baby. These findings are surprising and revolutionary: babies are more sensitive, more emotional, and more cognitive than we used to believe. Babies are not what we thought. In fact, babies are so different that we are obligated to create a new paradigm to accurately describe who they are and what they can do.[1]

Not long ago, experts in pediatrics and psychology were teaching that babies were virtually blind, had no sense of color, couldn't recognize their mothers, and heard only in "echoes." They believed babies cared little about sharp changes in temperature at birth and had only a crude sense of smell and taste. Their pain was "not like our pain," their cries not meaningful, their smiles were "gas," and their emotions not yet developed. Worst of all, most professionals believed babies were not equipped with enough brain matter to permit them to remember, learn, or find meaning in their experiences. [2]

These false and unflattering views are still widely held among both professionals and the general public. No wonder people find it hard to believe that a traumatic birth, whether cesarean or vaginal, can have significant consequences for life.

Unfortunately, today these unfounded prejudices still have the weight of "science" behind them, and babies are the victims whether the prejudices are old superstitions or new ones blessed by science. The resistance of experts who continue to see infants in terms of their incapacities may be the last great obstacle for babies to leap over before being embraced as the intelligent, capable beings they really are. Eventually, old ideas are bound to die under the sheer weight of new evidence, but not before millions of babies suffer unnecessarily because their parents and their doctors do not know they are human.

As the light of research reaches into the dark corners of prejudice, we may thank those contributing to the emerging interdisciplinary field of prenatal/perinatal psychology. Since this field draws from many types of scientific investigation and often requires collaboration, it does not fit conveniently into discreet academic departments and is not yet recognized in the academic world by endowed chairs or even by formal courses. At present only a few scattered courses in prenatal/perinatal psychology exist throughout the world. Yet research teams have achieved a succession of breakthroughs that challenge previous scientific ideas of human development.

Scholars in prenatal/perinatal psychology respect the full range of evidence of infant capabilities, whether from personal reports contributed by parents, revelations arising from therapeutic work, or from formal experiments. Putting together all the bits and pieces of information gathered from around the globe yields a fundamentally different picture of a baby.

The main way information about sentient, conscious babies has reached the public, especially pregnant parents, has been via popular media including books, movies, magazine features, and television. Among the most outstanding have been *The Secret Life of the Unborn Child*, a book by Canadian psychiatrist Thomas Verny (now in more than 25 languages), movies like *Look Who's Talking*, and talk shows like Oprah Winfrey, where a program on therapeutic treatment of womb and birth traumas probably reached 25 million viewers in 25 countries. Large circulation magazines like *Life*, *Time*, and *Newsweek* have featured cover stories on new discoveries about babies.

Four scholarly journals are now devoted to birth psychology. *The Journal of Reproductive and Infant Psychology* has been published in the United Kingdom since 1983. *The Journal of Prenatal and Perinatal Psychology and Health* began in North America in 1986, and the *International Journal of Prenatal and Perinatal Psychology and Medicine* began in Germany in 1989. To these must now be added the *Il Giornale Italiano di Psicologia e di Educazione Prenatale*, making its debut in 2002. Behind each of these scholarly journals is an official Association offering information to the public and high level educational

125

conferences to interested professionals.

Evidence that babies are sensitive, cognitive, and are affected by their birth experiences comes from various sources. The oldest evidence is anecdotal and intuitive. Mothers are the principal contributors to the idea of baby as a person, one you can talk to, and one who can communicate back as well. This process, potentially available to any mother, goes well beyond word-based language. This exchange of thoughts is probably telepathic rather than linguistic.

Mothers who communicate with their infants know that the baby is a person, a mind and soul, with understanding, sensitivity, and purpose. This phenomenon is cross-cultural and universal, since it can be found in the literature of all countries and regions of the world, through centuries of time--although all mothers may not actually engage in this dialog. In an age of "science," a mother's intuitive knowledge is too often discounted or dismissed. What mothers know has not been considered valid data. What mothers say about their infants is considered venal, self-serving, or imaginary, and can never be equal to the knowledge of "experts" or "scientists."

This prejudice extends into a second category of information about babies, the evidence derived from clinical work. Although the work of psychotherapy is usually done by formally educated, scientifically trained and licensed persons, the information they listen to is termed "anecdotal" and their methods are a blend of science and art. Thus, clinical evidence is not always accepted although the evidence of infant intelligence, based on the recollections of clients, is often compelling.

Therapists are privy to clients' surprising revelations that sometimes make a direct connection between traumas surrounding birth and later disabilities of heart and mind. Although it is possible for these connections to be purely imaginary, we know they are correct when confirmed by hospital records and eyewitness reports. Obstetrician David Cheek, using hypnosis with a series of subjects, discovered that they could accurately repeat the full set of left and right turns and sequences involved in their own deliveries. This is highly technical information that no ordinary person would have were it not for the memories themselves.[3] In my own work as a psychologist who started using hypnosis in 1974, I eventually found it necessary to test the reliability of memories people gave me about their traumas during birth, memories which had not previously been conscious. To do this, I hypnotized mother and child pairs who said they had never before spoken in any detail about that child's birth. I received a detailed report of what happened from the grownup child and compared this with the mother's report, given also in hypnosis.[4] The reports dovetailed at many points and were clearly reports of the same birth. By comparing one story with the other, I could see when the adult child was fantasizing, rather than having accurate recall, but my records showed that fantasy was rare. I concluded that these memories were real memories, and were a reliable guide to what had happened to the baby around the time of birth.

Some of the first clinical indications that babies are sentient came from the practice of psychoanalysis tracing back to the early 20th century and the pioneering work of Sigmund Freud. Although Freud himself was skeptical about the operation of the infant mind, his clients kept bringing him information which seemed to link their anxieties and fears to events surrounding their births. He theorized that birth might be the original trauma upon which later anxiety was constructed, although he persisted in believing these memories were fantasies.

Otto Rank, Freud's associate, was more certain that birth traumas underlay many later neuroses, and reorganized psychoanalysis around the assumption of birth trauma. For this he was rewarded by the rapid recovery of his clients who were "cured" in far less time than was required for traditional psychoanalysis.[5] In the second half of the 20th century, several important advances were made in resolving early traumas of womb life and birth.

Hypnotherapy, primal therapy, psychedelic therapies, various combinations of body work with breathing and sound stimulation, sand tray therapy, and art work have all proved useful in accessing important imprints, decisions, and memories stored in the infant mind. Had there been no working mind in infancy, of course, there would be no possibility of remembering anything and no need to heal bad impressions, change decisions, or otherwise resolve the mental and emotional problems associated with being born.

A third burgeoning source of information about the conscious nature of babies comes from carefully organized experiments and systematic observations utilizing new technologies. In Western culture, with its preference for refined measurement and strict protocols, these studies have become popular. Results are surprising from this contemporary line of empirical research. In truth, we have learned so much about babies in the last three decades that most of what we thought we knew before is suspect or obsolete. I will highlight this new knowledge in three sections: development of the physical senses, the beginnings of emotion and self-expression, and evidence of active mental life.

### Development of Physical Senses

First, we have a much better idea of our physical development--the process of embodiment from conception to birth. Our special interest is in the senses and when they become available to the fetus during gestation. Touch is our first sense, mediated by nerves which are built into the layers of the skin. Sensitivity can be measured in the face by about seven weeks gestational age (g.a.). Tactile sensitivity then expands steadily to include most parts of the fetal body by 17 weeks. In the normal womb environment, touch is never rough, and temperature is relatively constant. At birth, this placid environment ends with dramatic new experiences of touch that no baby can avoid.

By only 14 weeks gestational age (g.a.), the taste buds are formed and ultrasound shows both sucking and swallowing. A fetus controls the frequency of swallowing amniotic fluid and will speed up or slow down in reaction to sweet or bitter tastes. Studies show babies (and others) have a definite preference for sweet tastes. Recent studies have revealed the parallel function of taste and smell, now referred to as the chemical senses. Through constant exchanges between these senses in utero, babies are learning the taste and smell of their mothers and are well prepared to recognize and bond with them at birth.

Hearing begins earlier than anyone thought possible: at 16 weeks g.a. although the ear is not complete until about 24 weeks, a fact confirming the complex nature of listening, which includes reception of vibes through our skin, skeleton, and vestibular system as well as the various mechanisms inside the ear. Thus, babies in the womb are listening to maternal sounds and to the world outside the mother for almost six months prior to birth. By birth, their hearing is about as good as ours.

Our sense of sight also develops before birth, although eyelids remain fused from week 10 through 26. Nevertheless, babies in the womb will react to a light flashed on the mother's abdomen. By the time of birth, vision is workable but not yet perfect. Babies have no trouble focusing at the intimate distance between mother's breast and face, where the faces of mothers and fathers are usually found at birth. Newborns do not have to read microfilm or highway signs!

Mechanisms for pain perception are part of the sense of touch and develop early. By about three month g.a., if babies are accidentally struck by a needle inserted into the womb to withdraw fluid during amniocentesis, they quickly twist away and try to escape. Intrauterine surgery, a new aspect of fetal medicine made possible in part by our new ability to see inside the womb, provides new opportunities for fetal pain. Although surgeons have long denied pain in prenates, a recent experiment in London proved unborn babies do feel pain. Babies needled for intrauterine transfusions showed a 600% increase in beta-endorphins production, hormones generated to deal with stress. In just ten minutes of needling, even 23-week-old fetuses were mounting a full-scale stress response. Needling at the intrahapatic vein provokes vigorous body and breathing movements.[6]

Finally, muscle movement develops under the buoyant conditions in the fluid environment of the womb where muscles are regularly used in navigating the area. However, after birth, in the dry world of normal gravity, muscles look feeble. As everyone knows, babies cannot walk, and they struggle just to hold up their heads. Because muscles are still relatively undeveloped, babies give the appearance of incompetence. Except for the movement a mother and father could sometimes feel, we had almost no knowledge of the extent and variety of movement inside the womb.

This changed with the advent of real-time ultrasound imaging, giving us moment-by-moment pictures of fetal activity.

## Emotion and Self-Expression

One of the surprises is that movement commences around ten weeks gestational age. This has been determined with the aid of improved ultrasound technology. Fetal movement is voluntary, spontaneous, and graceful, not jerky and reflexive as previously reported. By ten weeks, babies move their hands to their heads, face, and mouth; they flex and extend their arms and legs; they open and close their mouths; and they rotate longitudinally. From 10 to 12 weeks onward, the repertoire of body language is largely complete and continues throughout gestation. Periodic exercise alternates with rest periods in utero reflecting individual needs and interests. Movement is self-expression and expression of personality.

Twins viewed periodically via ultrasound during gestation often show highly independent motor profiles, and, over time continue to distinguish themselves through movement both inside and outside the womb. Their movements express their individuality.

Close observation has brought many unexpected behaviors to light. By 16 weeks g.a., male babies are seen having their first erections. As soon as they have hands, babies are busy exploring everything available including feet, toes, mouth, and the umbilical cord; these are their first toys. By 30 weeks, babies have an intense dream life, spending more time in the dream state of sleep than they ever do after they are born.[7] This is significant because dreaming is a cognitive activity, a creative exercise of the mind. Dreaming is a spontaneous and personal activity.

Observations of the fetus also reveal a number of reactions to conditions in the womb. Such reactions to provocative circumstances is a further expression of selfhood. Consciousness of danger and maneuvers of self-defense are visible in fetal reactions to amniocentesis. Even when things go normally and babies are not struck by needles, they react with wild variations of normal heart activity, alter their breathing movements, may retreat from or attack needles, or even remain motionless for a time-- suggesting fear and shock.

In the womb, babies are alarmed by loud noises, car accidents, earthquakes, and even to a mother watching terrifying scenes on television. They swallow less when they do not like the taste of amniotic fluid, and they stop their practice breathing movements when their mothers drink alcohol or smoke cigarettes.

In a documented report of work with the fetus under ultrasound, a baby struck accidentally by a needle not only twisted away, but located the needle barrel and hit it repeatedly — a behavior suggesting anger and fear.[8] Similarly, ultrasound observers have reported seeing twins hitting each other, while others have seen twins playing together, gently awakening one another, playing cheek-to-cheek, and even kissing. Such scenes, some at only 20 weeks g.a., were never predicted in developmental psychology. No one anticipated social or emotional behavior until months after birth.

Emotion expressed in crying and smiling can be seen long before 40 weeks g.a. Smiles are first seen on the faces of premature infants who are dreaming. Smiles and pleasant looks, along with a variety of unhappy facial expressions, tell us dreams can be pleasant or unpleasant. Mental activity stirs emotional and physical activity. Audible crying has been reported by 23 weeks g.a. in cases of abortion, revealing that babies are experiencing very appropriate emotions at that time. Close to the time of birth, medical personnel have heard audible crying from within the womb, usually in association with obstetrical procedures that have allowed air to enter the space around the fetal larynx.[9] This shows that the capacity for baby crying is already developed before air is introduced.

### Active Mental Life

Finally, a further source of evidence for infant consciousness is research which confirms various forms of learning and memory in both the fetus and the newborn. Note that learning and memory are related: learning is not possible without memory; therefore, proof of learning is proof of memory. Because infant consciousness was considered impossible until recently, it has been hard for experts to accept a growing body of experimental findings showing that babies learn from their experiences. In studies that began in Europe as long ago as 1925 and in America in 1938, babies have demonstrated all the types of learning formally recognized and tested in psychology at the time: classical conditioning, habituation, and reinforcement conditioning, both inside and outside the womb.

In modern times, as learning has been understood more broadly, experiments have shown a full range of learning abilities. Immediately after birth, babies show recognition of musical passages which they have heard repeatedly before birth, whether it is the bassoon passage in Peter and the Wolf, the child song, "Mary Had a Little Lamb," or the theme music of a soap opera listened to frequently by their mothers.[10] Language acquisition begins in the womb as babies listen repeatedly to their mothers' intonations and learn their "mother tongue." As early as 28 weeks g.a., the recording of a baby's first cry contains so many rhythms, intonations, and other features common to their mother's speech that their elaborate sound spectrographs can be matched. In experiments shortly after birth, babies recognize their mother's voice and prefer her voice to other female voices. In the delivery room, babies can recognize their father's voice and react to specific sentences their fathers have spoken to them in the womb. After birth, babies show special acquaintance with their native language, preferring it to a foreign language.[11] Fetal learning and memory also includes stories that are read aloud to them repeatedly before birth. At birth, babies will alter their sucking behavior to obtain recordings of familiar stories. In a recent experiment, a French and American team had mothers repeat a particular children's rhyme each day from week 33 to week 37 g.a. After four weeks of exposure, babies reacted to the target rhymes and not to other rhymes, proving they already recognize specific language patterns learned in the womb.[12]

Newborn babies quickly learn to distinguish their mother's face from other female faces, their mother's breast pads from other breast pads, their mother's distinctive underarm odor, and their mother's perfume if she has worn the same perfume consistently.

Premature babies learn from their unfortunate experiences in neonatal intensive care units. One boy, who endured surgery paralyzed with curare, but was given no pain-killing anesthetic, developed a pervasive fear of doctors and hospitals that remained undiminished in his teens.[13] He also learned to fear the sound and sight of adhesive bandages—a direct reaction to having some of his skin pulled off with adhesive tape during his stay in the premature nursery.

Confirmation that early experiences of pain have serious consequences later has come from recent studies of babies at the time of first vaccinations. Researchers who studied infants being vaccinated four to six months after birth discovered that babies who had experienced the pain of circumcision had higher pain scores and cried longer. The painful ordeal of circumcision had conditioned them to pain and set their pain threshold lower. This is an example of learning from experiences of perinatal pain. Parents and professionals should be warned: pain is real and pain is damaging.

Happily, there are other things to learn in utero besides pain. The Prenatal "University" is a popular program of prenatal stimulation for parents who want to establish strong bonds of communication with a baby in the womb.[14] One of the many exercises is the "Kick Game," which you play by responding to the child's kick by touching the spot your baby just kicked, and saying "Kick, baby, kick!" Babies quickly learn to respond to this kind of attention: they do kick on invitation and can learn to kick anywhere their parents touch. One father taught his baby to kick in a complete circle.

Babies also remember the big event of birth itself. Proof of this comes from little children just learning to talk.[15] Usually around two or three years of age, when children are first able to speak about their experiences, some spontaneously recall what their birth was like. They tell what happened in plain language, sometimes accompanied by pantomime, pointing, and sound effects. They describe the womb water, darkness, redness, an increasing (or dazzling) light, and squeezing sensations. Cesarean babies tell about a "door" or "window" suddenly opening, or a "zipper" that opened the womb to let them out. Some babies recall their feelings of fear and danger. They also remember secrets.

One of my favorite stories of a secret birth memory came from Cathie, a midwife's assistant. When a home birth was completed, she found herself alone with a hungry, restless baby when mother had gone to bathe and the chief midwife was busy in another room. Instinctively, Cathie offered the baby her own breast for a short time, then wondered if this was appropriate and stopped without telling anyone what had happened. About four years later, Cathie was babysitting her. In a quiet moment, she asked the child if she remembered her birth. The child did, and volunteered various accurate details. Then, moving closer to whisper a secret, she said "You held me and gave me titty when I cried, and Mommy wasn't there." Cathie said to herself at the time, "Nobody can tell me babies don't remember their births!"

## Conclusion

Is a baby a conscious and real person? To me it is no longer appropriate to speculate about this--it is too late to speculate when so much is known. The range of evidence now available in the form of knowledge of the fetal sensory system, observations of fetal behavior in the womb, and experimental proof of learning and memory amply verifies what some mothers and fathers have sensed from time immemorial, that a baby is a real person. The baby shows intelligence in making creative efforts to adjust to or influence its immediate environment. Other signs of intelligence are seen in self-regulation (as in restricting swallowing and breathing), self-defense (as in retreating from invasive needles and strong light), and self-assertion, as in attacking a needle or doing battle with a twin!

Babies are like us in showing genuine feeling in reaction to assaults, injuries, irritations, or medically-inflicted pain. They smile, cry, kick in protest, manifest fear, anger, grief, pleasure, or displeasure in ways that seem entirely appropriate in relation to their circumstances. Babies are cognitive beings who think their own thoughts, dream their own dreams, learn from their own experiences, and draw conclusions from events. Because of all these proven abilities, we know today that babies remember their primal journey at a very deep level of consciousness. For better or for worse, they learn from the way they were received in the womb and the way they were treated at birth.

## References

1. Chamberlain, D.B. (1987). The cognitive newborn: A scientific update. *British J. of Psychotherapy,* 4(1), 30-71.

2. Chamberlain, D.B. (1991/1999). Babies don't feel pain: A century of denial in medicine. In *Selected Works of David Chamberlain, Journal of Prenatal and Perinatal Psychology and Health,* 14(1-2), 145-168.

3. Cheek, D.B. (1974). Sequential head and shoulder movements appearing with age regression in hypnosis to birth. *American J. of Clinical Hypnosis*, 16(4), 261-266.

4. Chamberlain, D.B. (1980/1999). Reliability of birth memories: Evidence from mother and child pairs in hypnosis. In *Selected Works of David Chamberlain, Journal of Prenatal and Perinatal Psychology and Health*, 14(1-2), 19-29.

5. Rank, O. (1924). *The trauma of birth.*

6. Giannakoulopoulos, X., Sepulveda, W., Kourtis, P., Glover, V., & Fisk, N.M. (1994). Fetal plasma Cortisol and b-endorphin response to intrauterine needling. *The Lancet,* 344, 77-81.

7. Roffwarg, H.P., Muzio, J.N., & Dement, W.C. (1966). Ontogenetic development of the human sleep-dream cycle. *Science,* 152, 604-619.

8. Birnholz, J., Stephens, J.C., & Faria (1978). Fetal movement patterns: A possible means of defining neurologic developmental milestones in utero. *American J. Roentology,* 130, 537-540.

9. Ryder, G.H. (1943). Vagitus uterinus. *American J. Obstetrics and Gynecology,* 46, 867-872.

10. Hepper, P. (1988). Fetal "Soap" addiction. *The Lancet,* June 11, 1347-1348.

11. Moon, C., Cooper, R.P., & Fifer, W.P. (1993). Two-day-olds prefer their native language. *Infant Behavior and Development,* 16, 495-500.

12. DeCasper, A.J., Lecanuet, J-P., Busnell, M-C., Granier-Deferre, C., & Mangeais, R. (1994). Fetal reactions to recurrent maternal speech. *Infant Behavior and Development,* 17(2),159-164.

13. Harrison, H. (1986). Letter. *Birth,* 13(2), 124.

14. Van de Carr, R.F., & Lehrer, M. (1997). *While you're expecting: Creating your own prenatal classroom.* Atlanta, GA: Humanic Trade.

15. Chamberlain, D.B. (1998). *The Mind of Your Newborn Baby* (3rd ed.). Berkeley, California: North Atlantic Books.

# DAVID HARTMAN, MSW
# AND DIANE ZIMBEROFF, M.A.

## MEMORY ACCESS TO OUR EARLIEST INFLUENCES

*An adult in hypnotherapy can age regress to a pre-episodic childhood experience, e.g., age one or two or the womb, and can nevertheless 'know' certain information about the experience. They know it to be true, without being capable of remembering it.*
*We explore how this phenomenon happens.*

~~~~~

David Hartman is a licenced social worker working in the USA, and editor of *The Journal of Heart-Centered Therapies*. Many archived articles are available free at www.wellness-institute.org.

Diane Zimberoff is a Marriage and Family therapist, also working in the USA and has been a speaker and hypnotherapy trainer since 1985. Author of *Breaking Free from the Victim Trap*, Diane has travelled to and trained professionals in Europe, Asia, Africa, and the Middle East since 1995.

*Extract from article published online in*
*Journal of Heart-Centered Therapies, 2002, Vol. 5, No. 2, pp. 3-63*

# 13

## MEMORY ACCESS TO OUR EARLIEST INFLUENCES

*David Hartman MSW
and Diane Zimberoff M.A.*

Practitioners of Heart-Centered Therapies and many other regression therapists have anecdotal evidence of the individual's ability to hypnotically follow an affect or somatic bridge back to memories at or near birth, or even earlier back to experience in the womb. Barbara Findeisen describes this situation aptly:

> Memories of early trauma are there, underneath the surface. They're there in our dreams, attitudes, even in our vocabulary. People unconsciously walk around in them all day but are not aware of where they come from. Many times after a birth regression clients say, 'I live this pattern every day. It never occurred to me that it might start that early.'[1]

Some people may ask, how is it possible that a prenate or newborn could process and understand experiences and create memories of them? And how is it possible that such memories, if they were created, could significantly affect that individual later in life? In this paper, we address these two fascinating questions.

First, let's assess documentation that the fetus and neonate do have sentient experience, and that they record the experiences in memory which is accessible later. Then we review current neurobiology research to trace the way in which early deeply encoded memories persevere over time and profoundly influence behavior in later life.

## Internal developmental influences

As early as 13 weeks gestational age, the fetus is showing individual behavior and personality traits that continue on after birth. Piontelli [2] observed four sets of twins by ultrasound periodically over the course of the pregnancies. Each set of twins seemed to manifest a unique relationship together: one set was loving, another contentious, and another was passive. One pair consisted of a brother who was active, attentive, and affectionate, and his sister who would passively follow his lead. The boy in this pair kicked and wrestled with the placenta, actively pushing for space and looking disgruntled. However, at times he would reach out to his sister through the membrane separating them, caressing her face or rubbing her feet with his. His sister would reciprocate when he initiated contact.

Piontelli conducted follow-up observation of the four sets of twins through age four. She found that behavior after birth for each child, and in the relationship between each set of twins, continued remarkably unchanged. The twins just mentioned continued to be affectionate with each other. At one year of age they would play together, touch, hug and kiss. The boy was self-starting and independent, and the girl passively followed his lead. The other twin pairs exhibited the same behaviors and relationship postnatally as they had in the womb. What accounts for the individual differences? One factor, of course, is the maternal environment in which each child lives. Another is its own genetic makeup. Could there be other factors that a child brings into the world - predispositions, prior agreements or commitments, or karmic debts? That question remains open for further investigation at another time.

By 20 weeks gestational age the fetus exhibits most of the movements that it will produce during its time in utero, and exhibits motor patterns similar to those observed in pre-term and term infants, including over 20 movement patterns.[3] It is well documented that fetuses dream, exhibited by rapid eye movement (REM), as early as 23 weeks gestational age.[4] Studies of premature babies reveal intense dreaming activity occupying 100% of sleep time at 30 weeks and gradually diminishing to around 50% by term.[5]

The dreaming activity, in both fetus and premature baby, is vigorous, involving apparently coherent movements of the face and extremities, and changes in heart rate and respiration, in synchrony with the dream itself. The dreams are, as with adults, expressions of inner mental or emotional conditions and are markedly pleasant or unpleasant.[6] While dreaming, babies exhibit their first smiles, and show their most frequent smiling in the dream state.[7]

The first breathing movements are observed [9] around weeks gestational age, and are regular in nature.[8] Of course, the fetus is unable to breathe in the fluid-filled uterus. Yet it makes movements of the diaphragm and rib cage that will result in breathing after birth. By 30 weeks, fetal breathing movements are episodic in nature occurring around 30% of the time.[9]

Anand and Hickey[10] specify the anatomical pathways and mechanisms for pain perception from the seventh week after conception onward. They point to the early origins of the neurochemical systems associated with pain, especially substance P, which appears in the brain and spinal column at 12 to 16 weeks. They note the consistent and predictable effect of prenatal pain on the cardio-respiratory system, on hormonal and metabolic changes, motor responses, facial expressions, crying and other complex behaviors including long term memory. The fetus responds reflexively to touch

141

around 8 weeks gestational age, and by 14 weeks most of its body (excluding its back and top of the head) is responsive to touch. The fetus responds to light with changes in body movements and heart rate from 26 weeks. The fetus' eye and body movements have settled into predictable patterns of behavior by 36 weeks gestational age, representing a greater degree of integration between the various centers of the central nervous system. Nijenhuis et al.[11] identified four 'fetal behavioral states' that are stable over time and observed repeatedly:

State 1: Quiescence, with only occasional startles; no eye movements; stable fetal heart rate.

State 2: Frequent and periodic gross body movements; eye movements present; fetal heart rate shows frequent accelerations in association with movement.

State 3: No gross body movements; eye movements present; fetal heart rate shows no accelerations and has a wider oscillation bandwidth than State 1.

State 4: Continual activity; eye movements present; fetal heart rate unstable and tachycardia.

The fetus is capable of discriminative learning, which requires some form of sentient awareness. Memory for prenatal experiences is present immediately after birth. For example, newborns prefer a lullaby their mothers had sung to them in the womb to an unfamiliar one sung by their mothers. [12,13] After birth, babies prefer to hear stories which were read to them in the womb, rather than unfamiliar stories.[14,15] Hepper [16,17] found that newborns of mothers who had consistently watched a particular television soap opera during pregnancy responded, when played the theme song after birth, by stopping crying, becoming alert, and changing their heart rate and movements. The newborns did not respond to other unfamiliar television tunes. Casper [18] says, "Human response to sound begins in the third trimester of life and by birth reaches sophisticated levels." Interestingly, Hepper found that the differential responding had ceased within 3 weeks of birth.

Prenates as early as 26 weeks learn intonations, rhythms and other speech patterns of the mother's voice, demonstrated in matching spectrographs.[19] By the age of 4 days after birth, infants can distinguish language from other sounds, prefer their mother's voice to that of another female, and prefer their mother's language.[20] They discern a language by its intonation and rhythm[21] and have done so with the mother's voice during the third trimester of pregnancy.[22] The prenate has already learned neural patterns of language, including the emotional context for phonological rhythms, tones and sequences of mother's speech. That is to say that at birth, French infants already understand that their language is syllable-timed, English infants understand that their language is stress-timed, and Japanese infants understand that their language is mora-timed.[23] These prenatal experiences are learning experiences, and are recorded in memory.

## Prenate awareness

Based on fetal observation and age regression findings, we can piece together a dim outline of prenatal awareness. This is highly speculative, of course; however, it is an experience all humans have shared, and on which there is a burgeoning body of research. There is no sense of self, identity or autonomy for the prenate. Rather, it lives in an undifferentiated state, identified with its environment, absorbing the mother's emotions and belief system as its own.[24] There is no sense of time, no reference to past or future. There is no defense against "negative" experience, i.e., the fetus is receptive and reactive to all experience, incorporating it into its growing blueprint of core beliefs. The fetus does eventually develop primitive defenses, or learned responses, in reaction to its experience, and in the process develops the beginnings of a self separate from the mother.

The prenates in Piontelli's study developed characteristic ways of being, e.g., contentious or passive or loving. These behaviors expressed an underlying belief system: perhaps "the mother/ environment is unreliable" leading to self-reliance, or to adaptivity, or to withdrawal; perhaps "the mother/ environment is toxic and confused" leading to powerlessness, or to oppositional reaction.

The fetus actually begins the process of moving away from total identification with the mother, and establishing a rudimentary ego differentiation that continues through adolescence. An example is a study[25] in which pregnant habituated smokers were forbidden cigarettes for several days. When the women were allowed to resume smoking, prenatal monitors detected immediate stress reactions before the mothers had actually lit the cigarettes. Although the mothers' thoughts and physiological anticipation were positive and pleasant, their fetus' reactions were distressed and negative. Not only were the prenates reacting to their mothers' anticipated experience rather than an already accomplished one, they did so with a personal point of view (distressed) rather than simply absorbing the mother's experience (pleasant) unfiltered.

Perhaps more bewildering yet, recent research seems to document that a newborn brings with it from the womb information not derived from sensory sources at all. One study[26] shows that only minutes after birth, babies can pick out their mother's face from an array of enlarged portraits.

These newborns' optic processing was so immature that their visual capability cannot explain the face recognition. Perhaps we need to keep an open mind regarding the existence in the prenate and neonate of a mind whose knowledge is not limited to its sensory experience, and whose memory is not limited to its central nervous system functioning.

## Function of developing systems precedes their completion

A vital fact about human development is that components of a biological system come into use before the system itself is fully functional. In fact, use is necessary for development to proceed. For example, the first heartbeat is at about 23 days after conception, long before the heart's valves, chambers, and blood vessels are completed. The sense of taste begins at about 14 weeks gestational age, and fetuses prefer sweet tastes over bitter and sour tastes (expressed through increased swallowing). The fetus' nose develops between 11 and 15 weeks, and while its sense of smell develops for use after birth with the advent of airborne odors, it tastes odors in the amniotic fluid with chemosensory receptors in the taste buds.

The fetus has access to an average of 120 odiferous compounds in utero, and learns to react to them.[27] A fetus is capable of behaviorally responding to sound at 16 weeks gestational age, long before the ear is structurally complete at about 24 weeks.[28] At 20 weeks, the fetus is sensitive to light, and twins are able to touch faces and hold hands, even though the eyelids remain fused closed until about the 26th week. The central nervous system is completed long after the fetus begins processing information, responding to it, and recording it in memory.

## Development of capacity to respond, remember, and make decisions

The unborn human develops the capacity to respond to the environment almost immediately upon conception. The central nervous system's limbic system is partially mature at 4 weeks of gestation and fully formed by the third trimester of prenatal life.[30] The limbic system records the emotions and behaviors necessary for survival, and is critically involved with the storage and retrieval of memory.[31] The cerebral cortex, the highest level of brain functioning, has been found operative by 32 weeks of gestation, [32,33] although it is far from fully functional. With the capacity to respond comes the ability to store experiences in memory for future use. Recent research [34] supports the capacity of the prenate to store very early traumatic experience in the bodymind (Pert's terminology), expressed permanently in psychosomatic conditions. The capacity to respond and remember carries with it, by definition, the ability to make decisions and choices.[35,36]

## Procedural and Implicit Memory

People generalize their experience into prototypes and rules, starting very early in life. The child, fetus or conceptus detects patterns and regularities in its environment and extracts them from the experiences themselves, forming "early conclusions" or "internal working models." These extracted generalizations are encoded and stored as implicit procedural memories: "Learning related to affect exchange within the attachment relationship is processed in procedural memory and is thus stored in an implicit manner."[37]

If the individual's early experience in relationships was unhealthy, toxic or aberrant, then they will proceed to extract unhealthy aberrant rules and generalizations: "garbage in, garbage out." Examples of implicit procedural memories are: "When I touch fire, it hurts." "I like the attention I get when I compete successfully." "Men are dangerous." These personal rules are not conscious, and the original events upon which they were extracted are not available to conscious memory for processing. It is important to realize that these memories and the resulting "knowledge" are not unconscious because of repression, defense, anxiety, or internal conflict.[38] They are unconscious because the brain system encoding them works at a level of awareness below consciousness. Nevertheless, they exert a profound influence on behavior over a lifetime by initiating reflexive reactions, i.e., "repetition compulsion" or "recapitulation" of early patterns.

Implicit memories determine behavior in a second primary way. These implicit memories, again unconsciously, "exert a self-perpetuating bias for interpreting later experience in a light consistent with past experience, whether later experience is objectively consistent with past experience or not"[39] This explains the phenomena of transference and projection. Emotional expectations which were validly learned in past relationships are transferred into present relationships without objective reality-testing for evidence of accuracy. Statebound learning occurs in young children, including the fetus, not just in traumas but in every experience, resulting in internal working models.

For example, fetuses of women with chronic stress have fast heart rates and are very active.[40] The fetus may experience that its mother's constant stress level is lowered, bringing calming relief, only when it also experiences nicotine or sugar or alcohol in the blood supply. This lesson is learned at the deepest layer of the developing fetus' nervous system functioning, and re-enacted unconsciously later in life in the compulsive self-medicating use of nicotine, sugar or alcohol. The memory is not verbal or conceptual, it is viscerally imprinted. The only means of accessing it for possible change is to return to the state in which it was learned: re-living the original experience as it was first experienced, then re-living it with a "corrective experience," allowing the option of consciously changing the outcome.

The repeated 'mini stress' involved in the therapeutic sensory and emotional reviewing of the traumatic event in hypnosis can partially reactivate the stress-released hormonal information substances that originally encoded that event in a statebound condition. The body actually remembers physical sensations and recreates these body memories during hypnosis age-regressions or other deep experiential transpersonal experiences. The statebound information is brought into consciousness, where the client's ordinary cognitive and verbal ego can process it. This allows the statebound or dissociated memories of the traumatic event, the basis of internal working models, to be accessed, processed, and therapeutically resolved.

~~~~~

## References

1. Mendizza, M. *Lifelong Patterns: Fear or Wholeness? Michael Mendizza Interviews Barbara Findeisen*. (Available at www.birthpsychology.com/lifebefore/early6.html.)

2. Piontelli, A. (1992). *From Fetus to Child*. London: Routledge.

3. Prechtl, H. F. R. (1988). Developmental neurology of the fetus. *Clinical Obstetrics and Gynaecology, 2*, 21-36.

4. Birnholz, J. C. (1981). The development of human fetal eye movement patterns. *Science,* 130, 679-681.

5. Chamberlain, D. B., & Arms, S. (1999). Obstetrics and the prenatal psyche. *Journal of Prenatal and Perinatal Psychology and Health,* 14(1/2), 97-118.

6. Roffwarg, H. A., Muzio, J. N., & Dement, W. C. (1966). Ontogenetic development of the human sleepdream cycle. *Science,* 152, 604-619.

7. Emde, R. N., Swedburg, J., & Suzuki, B. (1975). Human wakefulness and biological rhythms after birth. *Archives of General Psychiatry*, 32, 780-783.

8. De Vries, J. P. P., Visser, G. H. A., & Prechtl, H. F. R. (1985). The emergence of fetal behaviour II: Quantitative aspects. *Early Human Development*, 12, 99-120.

9. Patrick, J., Campbell, K., Carmichael, L., Natale, R., & Richardson, B. (1980). Patterns of human fetal breathing during the last 10 weeks of pregnancy. *Obstetrics and Gynecology*, 56, 24-30.

10. Anand, K. J. S., & Hickey, P. R. (1987). Pain and its effects in the human neonate and fetus. *New England Journal of Medicine*, 317(21), 1321-1329.

11.Nijenhuis, E. R. S., Prechtl, H. F. R., Martin, C. B., & Bots, R. S. G. M. (1982). Are there behavioural states in the human fetus? *Early Human Development*, 6, 177-195.

12. Satt, B. J. (1984). *An Investigation into the Acoustical Induction of Intrauterine Learning*. Dissertation, California School of Professional Psychology, Los Angeles.

13. Panneton, R. K. (1985). *Prenatal Auditory Experience with Melodies: Effect on Post-Natal Auditory Preferences in Human Newborns*. Dissertation, University of North Carolina, Greensboro.

14. DeCasper, A., & Spence, M. (1982). Prenatal maternal speech influences human newborn's auditory preferences. *Infant Behavior and Development*, 9, 133-150.

15. Woodward, S. C. (1992). *The Transmission of Music into the Human Uterus and the Response to Music of the Human Fetus and Neonate*. Dissertation, University of Capetown, South Africa.

16. Hepper, P. G. (1988). Foetal 'soap' addiction. *Lancet*, ii, 1347-1348.

17. Hepper, P. G. (1991). An examination of fetal learning before and after birth. *Irish Journal of Psychology*, 12, 95-107.

18. DeCasper, A. J., & Fifer, W. P. (1980). Of human bonding: Newborns prefer their mothers' voices. *Science,* 208, p.1174

19. Truby, H. M. (1975). Prenatal and neonatal speech, pre-speech, and an infantile speech lexicon. *Child Language* 1975, a special issue of WORD, 27, parts 1-3.

20. Mehler, J., & Christophe, A. (1995). *Maturation and learning of language in the first year of life.* In M. S. Gazzaniga (Editor-in-Chief) & S. Pinker (Language Section Ed.), *The Cognitive Neurosciences,* 943- 954. Cambridge, MA: The MIT Press.

21. Mehler, J., & Dupoux, E. (1994). *What Infants Know: The New Cognitive Science of Early Development* (P. Southgate, Trans.). Cambridge, MA: Blackwell.

22. Childs, M. R. (1998). Prenatal language learning. *Journal of Prenatal and Perinatal Psychology and Health,* 13(2), 99-121.

23. Otake, T., Hatano, G., Cutler, A., & Mehler, J. (1993). More or syllable? Speech segmentation in Japanese. *Journal of Memory and Language*, 32, 258-278.

24. Givens, A. M. (1987). The Alice Givens approach to prenatal and birth therapy. *Journal of Prenatal and Perinatal Psychology and Health,* 1(3), 223-229.

25. Lieberman, M. (1963). Early developmental stress and later behavior. *Science*, 141, 824.

26. Walton, G. E., Bower, N. J. A., & Bower, T. G. R. (1992). Recognition of familiar faces by newborns. Infant Behavior and *Development,* 15, 265-269.

27. Schaal, B., Orgeur, P., & Rognon, C. (1995). *Odor sensing in the human fetus: Anatomical, functional, and chemeoecological bases.* In J. P. Lecanuet, W. P. Fifer, N. A. Krasnegor, & W. P. Smotherman (Eds.), *Fetal Development: A Psychobiological Perspective,* 205-237. Hillsdale, NJ: Lawrence Erlbaum Associates.

28. Shahidullah, S., & Hepper, P. G. (1992). Hearing in the fetus: Prenatal detection of deafness. International Journal of Prenatal and Perinatal Studies, 4(3/4), 235-240.

29. Pert, C. (1987). Neuropeptides, the emotions and bodymind. In J. Spong (Ed.), *Proceedings of the Symposium on Consciousness and Survival*, 79-89. Institute of Noetic Sciences.

30. Pert, C., Ruff, M., Weber, R. J., & Herkenham, M. (1985). Neuropeptides and their receptors: *A psychosomatic network. Journal of Immunology*, 135(2), Supplement, 820-826.

31. Van der Kolk, B. A. (1996). *The body keeps the score*. In B. A. van der Kolk, A. C. McFarlane, & L. Weisaeth (Eds.), *Traumatic Stress: The Effects of Overwhelming Experience on Mind, Body and Society*. New York: The Guilford Press.

32. Purpura, D. P. (1975). *Normal and aberrant neuronal development in the cerebral cortex of human fetus and young infant*. In M. A. G. Brazier, & N. A. Buchwald (Eds.), *Basic Mechanisms in Mental Retardation*, 141-169. New York: Academic Press.

33. Vaughn, H. G. (1975). Electrophysiological analysis of regional cortical maturation. *Biological Psychiatry,* 10, 313-326.

34. Marquez, A. (2000). Healing through prenatal and perinatal memory recall: A phenomenological investigation. *Journal of Prenatal and Perinatal Psychology and Health*, 15(2), 146-172.

35. Hull, W. F. (1986). Psychological treatment of birth trauma with age regression and its relationship to chemical dependency. *Pre- and Peri-Natal Psychology Journal*, 1, 111-134.

36. Lake, F. (1982). *With Respect: A Doctor's Response to a Healing Pope*. London: Darton, Longman & Todd, Ltd.

37. Amini, F., Lewis, T., Lannon, R., Louie, A., Baumbacher, G., McGuinness, T., & Zirker-Schiff, E.(1996). Affect, attachment, memory: Contributions toward psychobiologic integration. *Psychiatry*, 59, 213-239.

38. Amini et al., (1996). ibid.

39. Amini et al., (1996) ibid. p. 228

40. Klaus, M. H., & Klaus, P. (1998). *Your Amazing Newborn*. Reading, MA: Addison-Wesley.

# NICK OWEN

## MYTHOLOGY AND THE WOMB TWIN

*Key Greek and Roman myths should leave us in no doubt of the importance of twins separated by death. They are at the foundation of some of our greatest civilizations. But the folk tales, theatre and literature of today continue to reveal the powerful psychological and emotional persistence of a dead womb twin in the world of the living. This study examines the psychology and meaning of some of these tales, in particular the Changeling story.*

~~~~~

Nick Owen is a poet, photographer, and guide through journeys of transformation. He has been a psychotherapist and director of the Oxford School of Psychotherapy and Counselling, working with and teaching about birth psychology for over thirty years. He now works for The Oxford Prenatal and Perinatal Education Research and Awareness Trust.

*An original, previously unpublished article*
*© Nick Owen 2006*

# 14

## MYTHOLOGY AND THE WOMB TWIN

*Nick Owen*

The insights of poetry leave science trailing behind. Samuel Coleridge wrote that the history of man in the nine months preceding birth would probably be far more interesting and contain events of far greater moment than all the three score years that followed it.

Research into the life of the womb twin survivor indicates that the life that follows birth is, to a significant extent, a recapitulation of the dramas that went on in those first months of life in the womb. This is one of the conclusions made by Ludvig Janus in his ground-breaking book, *The Enduring Effects of Prenatal Experience,*[1] which surveys the field of prenatal psychology from its beginnings to the present day.

The dramas we find ourselves living out in our lives are also translated into works of mythology, literature, art and folk or fairy tale. In this piece, I explore variations on one of these dramas, or themes: that of the Changeling. The changeling is a fairy replacement for a human baby, who is spirited away soon after birth. It is a story very widely known and repeated in the British Isles. It is also the most striking form of encounter between the world of the fairies and the human world. The changeling baby soon disappears itself. But why do humans need such a complicated and implausible explanation for the death of a baby? This piece will provide some level of explanation in terms of the existence of a womb twin, who remains very much alive in the psyche of the survivor.

Firstly, I will add a little about my own background.
I am a womb twin survivor. The need to restore the intimate
Other I knew in the womb has been the key motivator in my
becoming a psychotherapist. My first qualification was as a
drama teacher. I also trained as a Jungian psychotherapist,
social group-worker, and psychodramatist. I began using
myths and fairy tales in personal development workshops
in 1976. I have done this for over thirty years now, helping
people to make sense of their personal and family stories;
helping them grow into more mature human beings; making
therapeutic changes in their lives. The fairy tale workshops
have always started with a dramatic re-enactment of a tale
by a small group of people aged from sixteen to ninety nine.
We then explore the meaning of the story and its relevance
to the teller's and other group members' lives.

As with all depth psychology, the more you discover
the deeper you go. Going deeper often means going closer
to the root of things; to the beginning of time and life, never
forgetting that it is what is alive now that really counts.
It is a bit like removing the layers from a Russian doll.
One pattern has another similar but subtly different pattern
underlying it. The deepest layers were impenetrable to the
psychoanalysts. Even Jung did not believe that there could
be a personal history, as opposed to an archetypal pattern
of learning, before birth. Jung thought that myths and fairy
tales reveal the fundamental structures of human thought,
much as Plato believed in the existence of the "Forms."
This is true to some extent but it is not the whole story.

Not quite satisfied with Jung and Psychoanalysis
after five years of my own learning, I moved on to Primal
Psychology. Otto Rank took things further than Jung when
he wrote about the place of personal birth trauma in the life
of the individual.[2] But even birth is not the start of conscious
life. Intensive training workshops with William Emerson in
the 1980's revealed to me that personal trauma can begin at

conception, or in the process of becoming a twin, as well as in the subsequent loss of one of the twins.[3]

My thesis is that the child who loses a twin at the prenatal or perinatal stage of development becomes part human, part fairy. Put another way, descriptions of our encounters with the fairy world are a projection of our lost womb life.

The stimulus for this piece came from a programme on BBC Radio 4 called *In our Time* on Fairies.[4] This series explores our world history and culture through a weekly discussion of a particular subject. Until that moment, I had never thought of placing "fairies" alongside Freud, Jung, Evolution, the Heart, or Carbon as key foci for the history of our culture. Yet they do belong there. They have been important in many periods and in numerous cultures.

## The fairy

From this programme I learned that the first partner for Adam in Hebrew culture is not Eve, but Lilith. She transforms into a fairy. This primal model of a woman, having failed the requirements of the Hebrew God, is replaced by Eve in the Garden of Eden, and becomes a tormenting spirit, a fairy, who plagues women bearing children and blights their offspring. In fact, the Hebrews probably borrowed her from an even earlier Sumerian figure with the same characteristics. The fairy belongs in a parallel world, on the human level, not human, having special non-human powers, but not with the power of a God or Higher Being. They also have a special area of concern: loss, suffering, disappearance and death.

## The dead twin lives on

I find that the idea of fairies fits beautifully into making sense of the weird continuation of the dead twin in the life of the living one. It is the changeling story which best illustrates the ghostly continuation of the twin. It comes from relatively recent western folklore. Fairies are immortal like the Gods, yet they yearn for mortal life. Very old, they desire the company of the very young mortal; the new born human child. To this end, they often steal in to the human world at the time of a birth, and slip away with the new born baby, leaving in its place one of their own, looking identical to the child, yet with a highly developed intelligence, which humans can reveal and expose by trickery. (Parents of the womb twin survivor often comment that they think the child is otherworldly or unworldly. The child herself tends not to feel at home in this world. Whether any of this relates to the New Age *Indigo Children* phenomenon I will not speculate here.) The fairy impostor fades away in time, usually after a few months, leaving the human family bereft. By then it is too late to reclaim the real child from the fairy Kingdom under the hills.

In the BBC programme on fairies, it was suggested that changeling stories were probably part of an excuse for infanticide. Mortality rates at birth are always higher than any other time, however. With one twin dead around the birth time or before then, the second twin's chances of surviving are much reduced. Starting life as a twin is a massive risk factor for real time and later medical and psychological distress. That wicked fairy hovers a lot longer over the crib of a surviving twin. There are a number of cultures where one twin is killed at birth for religious reasons, and where a culture can not cope with this kind of confusing of identity.

The social anthropologist, Victor Turner, describes this in his book, *The Ritual Process* [5] but I have not seen evidence that a changeling diagnosis has been a general reason for infanticide. It is much easier in western cultures to call the unwanted child "devil's spawn" than a fairy.

## Snow White

The wicked fairy is the exception rather than the rule. Snow White is very likely to be a womb twin survivor however. The adult assault by the wicked Queen is more likely to be a pre-birth abortion attempt, recapitulated at puberty, as Ludwig Janus has explored in his seminal book on the enduring experience of life before birth. We can very usefully explore Snow White further in terms of attempted abortion. The three attempts by step mother to kill the girl in the forest may be three attempts by a mother to kill her unborn baby, with or without the help of a crone abortionist. The appearance of the helpful dwarves may prefigure the psychoanalytic discovery of splitting as a defence against traumatic invasion. One version of the tale actually has two girls, Snow White and Rose Red. The description of the special girl as "white as snow and red as blood" may be as much about death as beauty. I have written elsewhere of a psychodramatic exploration of this theme at an international prenatal and perinatal congress. [6] Sometimes the abortion kills one twin leaving the other to survive into adulthood.

## Roots of modern changeling stories in Greek Myth

Bettelheim, in *The Uses of Enchantment* [7] makes a distinction between the familial, domestic scale of the fairy tale, as opposed to the cosmic, grand scale of mythology. He thinks myths belong with whole cultures and society in general, while the fairy tale simply describes family dynamics. It is certainly better to stay with the domestic scale of things when unearthing personal history in a therapeutic group. But I find the Bettelheim distinction too simplistic, since many classical Greek myths are full of all-too-human domestic conflicts, spiced up by the activities of Gods that are themselves all-too-human in their morals and emotions.

The Greek twins, Castor and Pollux, are the pair most strongly associated with the astrological Gemini figure. The twin stars bear their names in the sky above us. They were the sons of Leda, the wife of King Tyndareos of Sparta. Zeus had turned himself into a swan to court his human object of desire. She, in turn, had changed into a swan trying to escape him. She laid two eggs as the outcomes of her mating with the God and with her husband. One egg held mortal children, Castor and Clytemnestra, the other the immortal children of Zeus, Pollux and Helen. The story continues with a struggle between the grown up Castor and Pollux and another pair of twins. During the fight Castor hides in a hollow tree, but is spotted there and killed by one of the other twin's arrows. Pollux is overwhelmed by the loss.

The grief of this twin survivor was so intense that even Zeus was moved to pity. He agreed that they could be reunited, spending half their time in heaven, half in the post death realm of Hades. So it is; they alternate between the poles of heavenly light and hell's darkness. This mortal-immortal split repeats over and over again in classic myth.

The story of Narcissus really deserves its own book. Much of Freud would need reworking if we took seriously the possibility that there is a real Other at the heart of this story. It will have to suffice to say that he fades away, like the changeling, absorbed completely in his lost mirrored Other, and mourned by an echo, a real world Other he cannot connect with. How many human marriages retell this story?

## The twinned culture hero

A significant number of ancient cultures are based on a twinning at the centre of things. The Spartans had twin Kings, one backing up the other. But while the Spartan warrior culture is based on a connected, collaborative twin relationship, the Romans experienced the competitive survivor struggle between twins. I would suggest the ruthless nature of their military empire/culture is based on this patterning. One story goes that Romulus and his friends killed and chopped up twin brother Remus into small pieces, which were smuggled secretly away. They then explained that Remus had mysteriously ascended to the divine realm without trace. This is more interesting for us than the usual tale of a fight over wall/ building, which is to say boundary making. It is an explanatory mythic story giving us a way of construing the disappearance by absorption of a twin lost in the early states of gestation.

Roman culture thrived on this kind of ruthless aggressive survival drive, while the Spartans also succeeded, but through their intense twin collaboration. There are dynamics of both collaboration and survival struggle in all twin relationships, with a great range of variation in any particular example. I believe all identical twin survivors have, to a greater or lesser extent, the swing between the poles of elation and depression, oscillation between Heaven and Hell. The hidden key to understanding the confusion and distress of a womb twin survivor is that they do not always know if they are the live Alpha twin or the ghostly changeling fairy. Both identities continue to exist connected with the survivor body.

## Shakespeare's Changeling story

So much of Shakespeare is an exploration of the lost and rediscovered twin. But one of his plays, the only one where he has not stolen the plot from someone else, is a play centred on a changeling. Midsummer Night's Dream describes the comic chaos which ensues when the King and Queen of the fairies fall out over possession of a changeling baby that Titania has taken from its mother, and will not relinquish to her Lord. Shakespeare fathered twins himself and may well be a survivor himself. His work is filled with lost and rediscovered twins. But only in this one play do we

meet a changeling at the very centre of the plot.  All of nature
becomes distorted when the changeling is misplaced.  Things
are not set right until Titania gives up her charge.  The
severe disturbance in vision, which the surviving twin often
experiences at the death of the other in real life, is at the very
heart of this play.

## The modern day changeling

A few years ago I found a children's story, outlining a very
informative version of the changeling motif, which echoes
very strongly the classic patterning.  An old couple are
delighted to have a child after many years of childlessness.
But they foolishly leave the new baby in the care of a family
pet.  While the pet sleeps, the little people come to the house
and steal the baby.  Much of the tale is then spent on how the
family pet atones for its sins by going into the underworld
to reclaim the child.  We need not concern ourselves with
the details of this heroic adventure.  What is important is the
resolution.  After living with the child for many months, the
Fairy King and Queen would be as bereft as the humans if
they were to lose the baby.  A witch from the upper world
adjudicates on the matter.  The child is to return to the human
world, but the baby is to spend part of the time with the
humans and part with the fairies.  Many motifs can be found
here.  The one that concerns us is the dual nature of the child.
It belongs in both worlds, human and fairy.  It is attached to
both worlds.  A higher power intervenes to create a resolution
which parallels the Castor and Pollux myth.

## The Once and Future King

Ted Hughes has written the most awesome of modern
changeling stories, *Gaudete*.[8]  In his story, an English
priest is taken into the hollow hills by the little people and
transformed into his double, who comes out to wreak havoc
on an English village.  Rather than explore Hughes' poetic

insights from Gaudete, I will pick up the Arthurian themes he draws on which reach back into antiquity and forward into the therapeutic journey some of us need to make in healing our womb twin experience.

The realisation that the dead twin "survives" and plays a key role in the psychological life of an individual is perhaps the most disturbing yet important discoveries I ever made as a therapist. Yet the most beloved of all stories outside of religious texts provides us with guidance, for the Grail Myths are full of womb twin imagery. The quest for the Grail is a story of coming back to ourselves, of reconnection with who we are. The Grail King has his shadowy twin, the Fisher King. The Grail quest is about reintegrating them. (Some would say that it is the Grail King who is the shadow.)

The main heroes who are sent out on the Grail quest, Percival and Lancelot, also fight with their inner other selves. *Parzival* [9] tells it something like this:

> *I mourn for them, these, the sons of one man. It barely makes sense to speak of two, for the two are one in body. Yet contending from good heartedness, flesh to flesh, blood to blood, was doing itself much harm.*

For those more interested in film than literature, one of the most memorable scenes in John Boorman's film *Excalibur,* [10] which attempts to follow the Mallory story, is the fight between Lancelot and his ghostly double. Lancelot dreams he is attacked by his double dressed in his armour. He wakes to find his own sword piercing his side.

### The Fisher King and the Grail King

I conclude with a telling of the Grail story interlaced with womb twin interpretation.

> *King Arthur is in his prime. He has apparently vanquished all his foes, and reigns over a Kingdom*

*thriving and at peace. Yet suddenly and mysteriously he is found wounded so deeply by a spear in his groin that it seems he cannot live...*

The land is laid waste as a result of King Arthur's collapse into the Beta twin identity, the changeling state. When there is a life crisis in which primal energies are disturbed there is the possibility of great suffering and great transformation. The journey of self discovery that is the Grail Quest is a tough road indeed. As each life change or transition is reached by any of us, the dynamics of our primal patterning will re-present themselves as new challenges, creating new problems and new opportunities for learning and deepening our understanding of life. Arthur has come to the throne young. He has triumphed over the young man's challenges. But faced with the challenge of inner relatedness, the deeper psyche, the lost twin, he needs help.

*Arthur becomes a changeling. He is a shadow of his former self. Somehow he hangs on to life. Perhaps it is the fairy, Morgan Le Fey, who has enchanted him, leaving him neither alive nor dead, neither fully in the spirit world, nor effectively in the land of the living. With the King so wounded the Kingdom itself starts to fall apart. There is climate change, famine, and drought. The people despair of the future.*
*Hope fades. Then a vision of the Holy Grail appears. Arthur announces that he will be restored if the Grail can be found in the real world and brought to him so he can drink from it. All the greatest knights of the realm are sent forth on the quest to find the Grail.*

The outer world is a reflection of what lies within. To heal the primal wound of inner conflict we naturally turn outside ourselves. This is the origin of the psychoanalytic term "projection". The vision of the Grail represents inner emotional healing. Arthur remains lost in the unresolved pain and conflict which comes from his origins. He calls on all of us to heal the world by healing ourselves.

*One by one all the knights are defeated. They either die on the quest or return empty handed. Yet even the strongest knight, Lancelot, fails this test. As in fairy tales, it is the youngest, the dumbling, Perceval, who is left alone to pursue the quest. We need not concern ourselves with all the details of Pereceval's many adventures on the journey. We catch up with him coming to rest one day by a river bank. A little further along the bank, he sees someone fishing. Who can this be?*

This is another representation of the wounded King, another Arthur, deeply wounded and unable to pull himself away from suffering.

*Perceval approaches the man, and asks him where he may find somewhere to stay for the night. The man is clearly injured and in pain as he sits by the river bank, holding on to his fishing rod. He replies that there is nowhere to stay for twenty miles. However, he has a place himself across the river just around the bend, if the knight can find it. Perceval accepts the kind offer and sets off along the river bank. But the landmarks begin to shift. The landscape becomes unfamiliar. Suddenly, a castle comes into view on the other side of the stream. As he approaches, a drawbridge is lowered allowing him to enter. Now he discovers himself to be in the Grail castle. Later the Fisher King appears and invites Perceval to dine with him. That evening, a great banquet is served and the four great treasures of the land are paraded before the amazed knight.*

*All drink from the sacred Grail except the Fisher King. He will not drink. He explains that his wound is*

*too deep. Not even the Grail can restore him to health,
or so he says.*

The Fisher King is lost in his own primal pain. The twin
has gone in reality, but he holds on to the pain of loss as if it
were ever present. He cannot escape from this state without
help from outside himself.

*The Grail is then brought before Perceval. But the
cup bearer asks him a question before he can take the
cup in his hands. "Who does the Grail serve?" says
the stranger. Perceval gives no answer. His courage
suddenly deserts him. He is overawed. His world swims
before him. He goes unconscious. When he wakes the
castle has gone. He is lying near his grazing horse by
the river bank. There is no sign of castle or Fisher King.
The Grail is no more than a brief memory.*

Perceval is overtaken by his own Beta twin self. Suddenly
he switches. In the Boorman film his life hangs by a thread,
a noose around his neck. To answer the Grail question he
must know he is both Alpha and Beta, and how to relate the
two. He must know himself more deeply than Arthur or the
Fisher King. But at this stage he does not.

*There will be years more of wandering, fighting,
learning, meditating, maturing his soul, before
another opportunity to encounter the Grail comes to
him. Beginner's luck or beginner's mind had brought
him early to the brink of success. But it had not been
enough. He had to develop wisdom. Some of that
wisdom comes to him after a battle with a Turkish
knight, whom he kills in combat, only to discover that
this is really his true brother. The foreign knight's
marbled skin reveals him to be a chimera, a being with
two people's entwined genes.*

In truth he has killed his own twin. The discovery of this
tragic womb twin loss begins his deepening process, but does
not in itself heal him.[11] The heroic way of the young man
is to overcome obstacles by Ego will alone. But that will
never win us the Grail. A much deeper wisdom is needed,
which comes from inner relatedness, relating to our inner
Otherness.

> *Many years of exploits go by. At last Perceval finds*
> *himself on the threshold of that other country, another*
> *world, once more. He crosses that draw bridge once*
> *more and is greeted by the Fisher King once more.*
> *A second time the banquet is set. A second time the*
> *four treasures of the land are brought forth. Once more*
> *the Grail bearer steps forward and asks the question.*
> *Perceval is now ready.*
> *"Whom does the Grail serve?" comes the question.*
> *"The Grail King," is Perceval's reply.*
> *At this moment everything changes. The Fisher King*
> *has gone. In his place emerges the Grail King in all his*
> *splendour. Perceval takes the Grail and offers it at the*
> *feet of the Grail King, who bids him drink from it.*

The Grail King is not simply the discovered other twin.
He is surrounded by all the symbols and mysteries of the
mythic world. It is not enough to know of another self.
The work for Perceval has hardly begun till he finds his
other, weaker self. The work of the Grail Quest is to bring
an integration of these understandings into a working reality.

> *Perceval has won the Grail. He takes it back with him*
> *to Arthur, his King, but as he returns to Arthur's court*
> *he witnesses the land itself is healing. The crops are*
> *growing again, rain falls, the sun shines gently down.*
> *Home at last, Perceval is not surprised to find that the*
> *work of the Grail is already done. Arthur is well again.*

This clearly shows us the profound relation between inner and outer worlds. The crisis and pain of discovery of the twin loss wound can lead into the half life of the wounded King. But it creates the possibility of a much deeper healing, a much deeper understanding of life. Jungians have analysed the relation between Fisher King and Grail King as that between Ego and Self. This interpretation is more direct and challenges some Jungian ideas about *shadow* and *animus/anima*. Perceval meets his first opportunity for transformation at the start of adulthood but he is not ready. He does not get another chance till a mid-life crisis point.

The key to Perceval's emergence as a true Grail winner and spiritual master is his realisation of the unity of the Alpha and Beta twin and a healthy relationship between them. At first he cannot cope with the challenge at all. Then he has tried to kill off his twin in the typically egoic, heroic, even Herculean manner. It remains indestructible, however many opponents in the outside world he conquers. Eventually he comes to an understanding of his own dual nature as he uncovers the true identity of the Fisher King. Indeed he has discovered that Arthur too has fallen into identification with the dead, yet still surviving twin.

At the first encounter inside the Grail castle he falls into the Beta state himself at the crucial moment and goes unconscious. The opportunity is lost. The second time around he is ready to grasp the Grail as the healing link between the two Kings, the two twins, Alpha and Beta, living and fairy.

Go find your Grail.

~~~~~

# References

1.  Janus, L.(2001) *The Enduring Effects of Prenatal Experience.* Mattes Verlag

2. Rank, O. (1929) *The Trauma of Birth.* London, Routledge

3.  Emerson,*W. Collected Works Vols 1 and 2. (*Privately published. Only available by personal application to the author.)

4. Bragg, M. (2006) *In Our Time: Faeries.* BBC Radio 4, May 2006

5. Turner,V. (1964) *The Ritual Process.* Penguin

6. Owen, N., (2002) *The Search for the Beloved.* Unpublished paper.

7. Bettelheim, B. (1975) *The Uses of Enchantment: The Meaning and Importance of Fairy Tales.* Vintage

8. Hughes, E. (1977) *Gaudete.* Faber and Faber

9. *Parzival* was an epic poem written in the late 12th century by the German poet Wolfram von Eschenbach.

10. *Excalibur.* (1981) A film directed by John Boorman. Warner Brothers

11. You can find much more about this story in *Occidental Mythology: The masks of God.* by Joseph Campbell (Penguin, 1976)

## Further reading:

Houston, J. (1987) *The Search for the Beloved.* Tarcher Putnam

Jung,E., Von Franz, M-L. (1970) *The Grail Legend.* Coventure

# THE JOURNEY TO IXTLAN

The journey to Ixtlan

begins

with the fearless
and profusely mythic story
of a return ... to somewhere...

one

... has never left,

...and

where we are always

leaving from....


*Anna Ruiz*

~~~~~

*Ana is a poet living in Parma, Ohio, USA. She posted this
poem on the Yahoo wombtwin forum in 2006, and it seemed
to describe very well the mysterious journey that it seems we
all must make towards self-understanding.*


*© Ana Ruiz 2006*

# PART FOUR

# THE PSYCHOLOGICAL
# EFFECT ON THE SURVIVOR

# TRACEY WILLIAMS

## WHEN HALF YOU IS MISSING

*Before Tracey found her wombtwin, she had spent her life racked with survivor guilt. She was slowly and compulsively starving herself to death. This is the story of how she discovered her lost twin brother, given in her own words.*

~~~~~~

Tracey is a professional journalist living in Hertfordshire, England.

*An original, previously unpublished article*

# 18

## WHEN HALF YOU IS MISSING

*Tracey Williams*

### Fat chance, slim hope

*Anorexia is like a drug. Inside my head is a little persistent voice saying, "Don't eat, don't eat." I won't. I feel good, I'm on a high. I've been good today, I've only had an apple. That's not perfect, I need to be better. Tomorrow, I'm not going to eat that apple.*

*Now I feel a failure. I shouldn't have done it today. Tomorrow I will be perfect. I will escape criticism. A tear trickles down my face. I feel lost, desperate. I need to get rid of it. I have failed again. How can I be successful if I constantly give in like this? I pace the floor, debating the best way to rid myself of it. A handful of laxatives or self induced vomiting? I choose both. I feel better now. Tomorrow will be better. I have learnt a hard lesson today. I have failed. I will be perfect and in control. I am in control now. I hide from others. They don't understand, they don't understand the complexities in my head. Faceless people get involved and my head is in turmoil. Now there are two voices fighting in my head.*

*"Eat, its good!"*

*"Don't eat! It's better!"*

*The argument is getting louder and louder. Where did it all go wrong? I shut my eyes and cover my ears.*

*"Go away, go away!" I scream silently.*

*I want it all to stop. I can't tolerate the arguments, the frustrations, the lack of control and more than anything,*

*the overwhelming feeling of defeat that constantly*
*surrounds me. However much I starve and vomit, it is*
*never enough. I want it to stop and yet I don't, because*
*then I will never achieve. Achieve what, I don't know,*
*but I will when I get there. Won't I?*

### The problem

Defeated and frail with pressure from these faceless
nobodies, I had to face the reality that I had a problem.
In my head it was only small. I wasn't going to die, just
achieve everything I always felt I had to. I had to regain part
of me. To everyone else, I was ill and without help. I was
going to die. I was 19 years old.

Finally and reluctantly I sought help. The pressure I
had put on myself was unbearable. I couldn't take it any
more. I wasn't achieving what I wanted to achieve. I felt a
failure, more so for seeking help. Starving hadn't worked
but I couldn't stop. I felt that perhaps I should stop but that
smacked of failure too. I didn't know where to turn, or what
I should do. I wanted to be a little girl again where there
were sunny days and Mummy and Daddy were there to tell
me that everything was OK.

I cried. I cried many times. All I could feel was despair.
They told me that the problem "wasn't insurmountable."
Try being in the head of an anorexic. It takes hold and grips
like an iron fist, refusing to let go and I didn't want it to.
However despairing I was, I felt strangely safe. For the past
five years, this had been all I knew. If this was taken away
from me, what would I have left?

### Anguish

I still convinced myself that I could stop, and I would, when
I got to where I had to be. I failed to recognise that that
place would be in a cemetery, only surviving in the memories
of those who cared about me. I had left nothing to the world

172

and nothing tangible of me would be left. I would only be a
memory that would gradually fade and die too.

I convinced myself that I was happy, but I would be
happier when I got there. If only I knew what that place was.
"I am in control", I told myself. "I will stop."

The anguish showed in the haggard faces of my parents.
My only concern was them. I was convinced I was OK but
I needed to make them see, make them understand. I also
wanted to be left alone, to battle my demons in peace.

### Counselling

In this hope I agreed to counselling. I was 20 years old.
Everything from my sexual history to my childhood was
examined, all of which was unfounded, since my childhood
was idyllic and my sex life healthy.

Believing these possible problems could be contributory,
the counsellors concentrated on these, whilst my parents
went through months of hell. Was it them? They asked
themselves. The strain showed but in the hope of getting
their beloved daughter back they persevered, taking me to
endless doctors and consultations. Everything was to little
effect, since all possibilities that the so-called specialists
came up with were so far removed from my reality.

### Deceit

Despite my pleas that I was OK, I continued along the path
of self destruction. No one found my laxatives. I would hide
food and vomit when no one was around to monitor where
I was and what I was doing. I would starve myself until I
was almost passing out. It was agreed, with the advice of
specialists, that a good move would be for me to live alone.
It would give me the opportunity, whilst continuing with
counselling, to stand on my own two feet, and, without the
pressure of being watched I would regain much of what
I had lost. Looking back, what a foolhardy decision that

was! I bought my own flat, close to my parents. I loved them deeply and couldn't bear to be parted from them. Yes, I craved my independence but I wanted them there. I wanted to be where I felt safe and secure. I still wanted to be a little girl. I wasn't ready to grow up.

### *Obsession*

My misplaced joy on moving into my own home was not that I could do what I wanted when I wanted, or party all night if I chose. Instead it was the realisation that I wouldn't have to eat anymore and no one would know! I could starve and vomit in peace.

Rather than tins of food or furniture, the first thing I bought myself was a set of bathroom scales. They were my most treasured possession. They dictated my life and my moods. They gave me the will to get out of bed each day, just to see if I managed to loose another pound.

I would vomit several times a day, whether I had eaten or not. After each occasion I would weigh myself, even after every wee. I would even take out my earrings with the fear that they would make me heavier than I was. What weight I wanted to be I had no idea. But, rather than embrace the lowness of my weight, I would hide it with baggy clothing. I looked in the mirror each day. I didn't see the bones sticking out. I didn't see that my stomach was concave rather than flat. All I could see were rolls of fat that really shouldn't be there.

It finally took its toll and I was forced into a stricter regime of diet and counselling under threat of hospitalisation. I knew couldn't carry on like this. I was killing my parents slowly with heartbreak, just as I was killing myself with starvation. I was thin and weak with self abuse. My parents were grey-faced and haggard with the life I was giving them. What right did I have to inflict this pain on them? They gave me life, a life to be treasured, the way they treasured me. Yet here I was, throwing all the love they had ever given me, back in their faces.

Their love and support for me was unflinching. Any lesser people would have walked away, but not my Mum and Dad. They stuck with me through it all. I wasn't fighting the battle on my own any more. There were three of us in it now. If I was going to go down, they were coming with me and my love and admiration for them could not let that happen.

### The struggle to heal

I realised that if I wanted to live, I would have to adhere to everything I was told. Forcing myself to eat and not vomit was one of the biggest tests of character I have had to face. I became like a caged animal, hysterical, violent, scratching, hitting out. I would scream, shout, cry, slam doors and punch walls. Desperation got the better of me and occasionally I gave in.

Paradoxically, I began to feel as if I had failed yet again. The dominant character was failure, whichever way I turned. Ironically, I felt, by slipping back into my anorexic ways that I was letting them down. Not necessarily myself, but my parents. The more I felt I was failing, the more I slipped back to the safety of starvation. I didn't know any better.

I had lost any self worth that I had, so what was the point? Looking at my parents gave me the kick I needed whenever I slipped back. My love for them was all encompassing so I resolved to strive and strive again.

### First marriage

I married at 21 in the belief that all my problems would be over. Needless to say, the relationship didn't work. My then husband couldn't deal with life with an anorexic and the marriage foundered. He would lock me in the house, pin me down kicking and screaming, force feeding me. But my weight dropped further. I felt I couldn't breathe, suffocated, fighting for breath. Hyperventilation combined with severe panic attacks prevailed and my anxious parents carted me of to casualty. I was sent away with, "You're underweight, keep on Prozac and take this Valium."

Signed off from work, I became a zombie for three months and I couldn't walk without the aid of a stick. I didn't want to feel like this. I firmly believed that I was better off before, without medical intervention. My pleas that the drugs didn't agree with me fell on deaf ears and eventually I took myself off them. I felt alone and dejected. Eager to find happiness, I left the marital home. I was living alone again and things would get better.

### *A new relationship*
In time, I met the man who was to become my second husband. He knew from the start what was wrong and stuck by me. Dealing with the stress of a mucky divorce, my weight plummeted to six and a half stone. I was warned that if my weight dropped any lower I would be admitted to hospital where I would be monitored and force fed.

Finally though, I was in a happy relationship and I had a new counsellor who, through endless consultations, taught me to change my thought processes. I now realised that I was endlessly searching for perfection, trying always through every aspect of my life, to achieve. I learnt to lower my goals, rather than constantly trying to achieve 110%. I realised that this was an answer and possibly for the first time I was on my way to recovery. I began to gain strength.

Our wish to start a family was the driving force behind further rehabilitation and despite all the odds, with a little bit of help, I fell pregnant. I have never known such joy and that gave me the impetus to eat. After all, I reasoned, I wasn't feeding me, I was feeding my child. She was more important than any of my hang-ups about food.

My desire to achieve was now focused on having a happy and healthy baby.

### *My daughter*

My daughter has helped me more than she will ever know. Because of her, I remained on an even keel. I fought the demons in my head and fought myself daily. It wasn't easy but she was too important to let down. I brought her into the world but she gave me life too. She gave me a reason to live rather than commit a slow, drawn- out suicide. It was my beautiful daughter who stopped me lapsing back when my beloved father died and my husband walked out six months later.

It would have been so easy to slip back into my old habits but I persevered. Her grandfather had gone, so had her father, but she wasn't going to lose me too.

I adapted to life as a single mother and continued to run my own business. Three years on, I was tested again. Having not allowed myself to recover from the death of my father and the breakdown of my marriage, my business failed and I was in debt.

Gradually life took its toll on me, I could feel myself being dragged back down into the pit of despair and anorexia. My demons had returned with a vengeance and this time they wanted to win. I fought it. I screamed and clawed my way to try to avoid it all from happening again. Now I tasted failure again, along with the shame that I was succumbing to the ravages of my illness. The depression that sought to engulf me began to take its toll – a build up of years of dealing with my emotions, feelings of never being good enough, feeling incomplete and unsettled and, above all, feeling that I was different to everyone else. Despite my battle with myself, I knew I was descending back into the safe clutches of that destructive illness.

The little whispers were becoming louder and more

persistent in my head. Looking into the cherubic face of my daughter with her crystal blue innocent eyes, trusting me unfalteringly to love and protect her, I knew that this time I would seek help before anorexia got its evil grip on me again.

## Finding David

I booked an appointment with Althea Hayton. I left two hours later, simultaneously shell-shocked and elated.
For the first time ever, I felt as if someone understood me.
It was as if she was sitting inside my head, pulling out the threads of my tangled thoughts and rearranging them to make some sort of sense.

Meeting Althea led me to know more about myself than I had ever known existed. I understood my feelings and inadequacies and the reasons for the anorexia. I felt that finally, someone understood me, knowing how I was feeling, without thinking me 'odd.'

Expecting the usual questions and hypotheses that had followed me around for the past 13 years, I was amazed to find myself answering questions such as:

*Do you feel different to everyone else?*
*Do you feel that you are constantly looking for something?*
*Do you feel you are not whole?*
*Do you feel settled?*

My answers, beliefs and the way I live my life all strongly pointed towards being a wombtwin survivor. Having spent 34 years as an only child, I am sure I reacted with a fair amount of surprise, disbelief and cynicism. Even now I can remember saying rather scathingly, "Well, where is he then?"

Undeterred by my rather selfish reaction, Althea explained the theory behind her statement. As she did so, everything gradually changed from a rather blurry

impressionist view of my life to a clear and concise reason
as to why I had done everything I could to commit a slow
suicide over recent years.

### *In search of proof*

By the time I left her, I knew that everything she said fitted
and made sense. My last bit of proof was to come from my
mother. I needed to know about my mother's pregnancy
with me.

I discovered that Mum had bled during the first trimester
of her pregnancy to the extent that she believed that she
had miscarried and was no longer pregnant. She was sent
away from the doctor's with the explanation that "these
things just happen." Yes they do, but it is only now that
the truth is starting to emerge. The loss of a twin isn't
just an occurrence. It creates a myriad of emotions and
complications and can affect the future in ways beyond
normal comprehension, - sometimes with devastating effect.

In my case, my mother had just miscarried my twin,
leaving me alone, a perfectly healthy foetus, to continue
developing normally. As well as the apparent miscarriage,
my mother found my birth difficult, 12 hours of agony and
forceps. Contradictorily, my birth weight was larger than
average, added to which, for a single baby the placenta was
unusually large.

Hours of discussion ensued. We delved back into my
childhood and adolescence. I showed traits indicative of
being a wombtwin survivor. As a child I had an imaginary
friend and unexplained bouts of moodiness. I was prone to
tears without being able to explain why. In my case, many
incidents in my childhood could not be explained, at least
not until now. My imaginary friend was a little boy who was
always there with me. He knew everything.

In order to tell what gender my sibling was, we looked
at my characteristics, the way I dress and the way I live my

life. All are indicative of a strong male link. I also had a huge guilt complex, both as a child and as an adult. I would get dreadful butterflies and nerves in my stomach. I would feel that "something was wrong" somewhere or "something terrible" was going to happen, for no apparent reason. Nothing bad did happen at those times as far as I am aware. What I was actually doing was recreating the feelings that were conveyed by my mother when I was in the womb.

I was experiencing that same stomach churning feeling she felt on seeing the blood and believing in horror that she had lost the baby that she had longed for.

I was never convinced that I was loved. I had the most idyllic and loved childhood but on many occasions from childhood through adolescence to adult hood, I questioned and tested that love. My parents had to reinforce it. Later in life even my daughter had to reinforce it.

What I was missing was the love of my twin. Once he had been there but he left me. I came out into the world alone and that scared me. I had lost the first thing I ever knew and the first person that I had ever loved.

All my life I had been constantly searching and endeavouring to find happiness, attempting desperately to fill a void that was present but not entirely sure how, therefore trying everything. My whole past is indicative of that first loss – the devastation of anorexia, the failed relationships, the constant changes of career and homes, always changing tangible elements of my life, trying desperately to get what I wanted, but never actually managing to get there and never finding what I thought I wanted to find.

The desperation of striving to attain was immeasurable, always followed by the feelings of failure. Whatever I did was never good enough. In each of the many careers I have attempted, I would never achieve what I thought I should. Every time I felt I might be getting closer, my goal edged just that little bit further away. In anyone else's eyes, I probably exceeded expectation but to me it was never enough. The problem was that I didn't actually know what I wanted to achieve. I know now that this is down to the fact that I was searching for my brother. With the memory deeply buried, the surviving twin can spend years searching for that vital missing factor without ever really knowing what that is.

I spent 34 years fruitlessly searching – but for what? All it resulted in was the desperate feeling of frustration and failure. Unwittingly, I was using my eating disorder to punish myself for my sibling's death, reacting against the deeply buried guilt that I had survived but he had not. I was trying to reach perfection through my body - a perfection that I would never have attained, because perfection is being whole. Without my brother, "whole" is something I would never be.

### *A positive outcome*

My case will never be proved scientifically as all this happened 37 years ago in the generation before scans, but from research and the physical signs, it has been proved beyond reasonable doubt. The influence this has had in my life is ever present but now it's positive. I don't want to die, I don't want to be an emaciated emotional wreck. Admittedly, I still have the occasional "fat" days, but show me a woman that doesn't!

Those days are in control now, no worse than any other menstruating and healthy woman. I look back now on those days and think, well, if hadn't been for him, I might not be here at all. If he knew I was trying to starve myself to death, he probably wouldn't be that overjoyed with me - after all, his life was stolen away to give me the opportunity of life. He is now part of my life and we have called him David.

I feel as if all my years in the wilderness are over, I know who I am and understand my characteristics and I finally feel that I am now where I should be. The overwhelming relief I feel shows in my demeanour and I have never felt this positive. For 34 years, I had been carrying round the guilt that I survived, but my twin didn't. A combination of this revelation of my 'lost' past', sheer will power and resolve, I think that this time I have beaten it. I have now triumphed. Yes, I have had two broken marriages and numerous failures. More importantly, I failed to become a successful anorexic but if success means death then I want no part of it. I have managed against the odds to have a beautiful daughter, through whom I am living everything I missed out on. If I had been a successful anorexic, I would never have found the joy that motherhood has brought me.

For the first time in my life I am glad I failed, for this failure has brought me strength and life that I never knew I could have and with my new found knowledge I have learnt to live again. I now I recognize that failure IS acceptable and it is through those moments that we learn and we move forward. More importantly I have accepted that without David here, there will always be a part of me that is missing but that is not MY failure. It is a sad fact of life and all I can do is treasure the life that he allowed me to keep. Only now, knowing what happened, can I finally put him to rest and move on. For the first time in my life, I feel loved and complete. I feel as though he is standing behind me, wrapping his arms around me and holding me close, protecting me. Not a feeling I have had before but the best feeling in the world. My only regret is the pain I put my parents through and the fact that my Dad cannot see me now. I only hope he knows.

# A WART ON THE NOSE OF DARWIN

Am I the one who went away? Am I the one allowed to stay?
I am the one who's here alone. I am the one who must atone.
I am the one who wonders why. I am the one who cannot cry.

I know not if it was a crime or was it just a fact of time?
Was it ordained or was it sought, could I kill with just a
    thought?
I never felt it was an end. I never felt it could not mend.

The world was us and I was me and ever it was meant to be.
Together we would on and on, two separate and yet as one.
We never saw, we never touched and yet we occupied so
    much.
It was as if we were as me; yet also separate and free.

At first it was a blinding fear, a thunderbolt rapped at my ear.
You seemed not there, but that could not be, for always it
    was you and me.
I searched, I strained, I screamed your name and then the
    awful truth it came.
It was the end, it was all doom, but yet time went on and I
    was alone?
Why was I spared? Why had I lived? Why was I left alone?

I've searched the cosmos for a cure, a balm to sooth my pain.
I have to have a reason why, an answer painted in the sky.
Why was it so? Why was it me? Was I the maker of my
    doom?

Am I so bad? Am I so sad that nobody could stay?
Was I the cuckoo in the womb, pre-programmed to survive
    alone?
Was I a victim in a womb that evolution made a tomb?
Was it all just fate that left me alone to wait?

*© Richard Moore September 2006*

# JOHN JAMES

## THE VANISHING TWIN SYNDROME, AND THE TRAUMATIC REALITY FROM THIS LOSS

*We can remember what happened in the womb. As the loss took place during our very creation, and as the impact is totally imbued into the cellular structure of our bones and muscles, therapy needs to be experienced at the cellular level. We need full consciousness of the moment of death to dissolve the disharmony this has created. Though permanent clearing can be immediate, some roots will always remain – for we are that experience -  and can be transformed into many positive directions in life.*

~~~~~

Dr. John James is an Australian architect, builder, farmer, transpersonal therapist and medieval historian with a passion for discovery.  For 30 years he has been searching to understand the workings of the human psyche.
He founded the Crucible Centre in the mountains west of Sydney where he and his colleagues have discovered how to work positively and directly with the energy of the True Self we call soul, that creates us in the womb and has a profound influence on our lives thereafter.  Their clinical work has included more than fifty VTS clients.  This has opened an enormous window into the hidden life of the foetus, and explains the decisions made in the womb that have influenced every aspect of their lives.

*The Crucible Centre Pty Ltd.*
*Lawson's Long Alley, Hartley Valley, NSW 2790 Australia*
*www.cruciblecentre.com*
*© John James 2006*

# 16

## THE VANISHING TWIN SYNDROME, AND THE TRAUMATIC REALITY FROM THIS LOSS

*John James*

For the past twenty-five years doctors have been aware that in twin pregnancies one can die in the womb.[1] In the medical profession it is referred to as the Vanishing Twin Syndrome (VTS). When reading the many reports and papers that discuss this matter, only the mother or the newly born baby are referred to. Doctors are, quite naturally, concerned that the presence of dead tissue in the womb may affect the health of either mother or infant.

This matter has only recently been addressed in therapy. When we produced our reports in mid-2005 I searched the web and the university periodical indexes for information, but could find nothing on the impact of inter-uterine death on the adult life of the living twin. It was as if the baby brought nothing from the womb but its body - and therefore anything else could be left out of the picture.

I am a director of the Crucible Valley Centre, an institute that teaches Transpersonal Psychology in New South Wales, Australia.[2] Our approach is experiential, and includes deep personal therapy with all students. We have been finding through them that the 'disappearance' of a pre-natal twin was often having a profound impact on the whole of later life of the living twin. This was not in a few isolated cases, but in hundreds of clients. It was a possibility my teacher Elia Carisbrook had mentioned almost twenty years ago and that I discussed in my 1994 book *Notes to Transformation*.[3]

It was not until the issue kept on turning up that we realised how enormous it was – both in numbers and impact.

With my wife Hilary and our partner Marg Garvan we
gradually became more open to the possibility that such
a death could affect the deepest psychic structures of our
clients. We have now worked with more than fifty VTS
situations and, based on its occurrence among our clients, we
estimate it affects more than 25 percent of all conceptions.
However, this proportion of one-in-four may not be reflected
in the general population. It may be that the buried grief
from the loss of a twin companion may induce more
people to seek therapy than others. This would reduce the
apparent proportion.

How do we know when someone has lost a twin in the
womb? One of our modalities is sandplay. It is a technique
that will often show our needs and feelings very clearly. In
the sandplay room there are a thousand small objects on
shelves around the room. You place them in a tray filled
with sand. We help the client discover the message from the
unconscious contained in the arrangement. This invariably
tells you exactly what is going on in the hidden parts of
yourself.[4] Here is one example:

*Fred is a steady worker, yet without much sense of*
*achievement. He is constantly searching for a woman,*
*but cannot form intimate or lasting bonds. In the tray*
*he created a diagonal axis with an almond-shaped*
*mandorla marked in the sand. Along this axis he placed*
*in the middle a glass ball enclosing a skull; a fossil*
*on the right, and between them clasped hands. A little*
*goanna was placed on the fossil, which he described as*
*having the feeling of "soft and uncertain longing." The*
*cross points to the skull. In the session he remembered*
*that he had been told he had had a girl-twin that had*
*died well before his birth. The session deepened when*
*he identified with the goanna and the fossil, and himself*
*helplessly holding on to the departed sister. He felt he*
*was like a "dead fossil" without her. His inner 'centre'*

*lay in the white hands, clasping onto the female who had gone.*

As therapists, we had to drop our own agenda and adapt to the client's truth. The feelings he was experiencing were so profound that we knew it was not just a story, but something that was deeply embedded in Fred's psyche. We were convinced by the emotional coherence of his experiences, not by anything else. In the sandplay the objects used and their symbolic significance made the meaning pretty clear.

Yet we puzzled for a long time on how was it possible for a foetus, often barely more than a few weeks old, to have feelings in response to an event in the womb, and continue to bear those feelings into adulthood. In the first trimester when most twins die, the foetus has a spinal cord but the brain is still miniscule. Yet our clients were describing memories and feelings recalled from the first trimester of life with absolute clarity.

We began to notice that more than emotional memories were involved. There seemed to be another factor that we could not relate to the simple reactions we would expect to find at the foetal level. There were clear indications from our client's work in the sandtray and in energetic processing that the remaining twin was responding to the death in ways that could only be called intelligent. It was if the foetus was being presented with choices, and swung towards one or the other with such determination that it affected the whole of later life. It was a process that could only be called 'decision-making'. This is an adult concept, yet there has been no other way to describe the clinical evidence.

We are taught that it is not until the infant is born that mind and feelings respond to the environment. We are told that at birth the baby has an 'unformed' mind and is still a *tabula rasa*, an empty slate. It became obvious that this cannot be true. It is evident now, after so many years as therapists working every day with early experiences and traumas, that this is nonsense.

We have concluded that losing a twin is one of the most powerful events occurring in the womb. It takes place so early in the creation of the foetus that any response is set into the later physical and emotional development of the baby. The foetus has feelings and its development is affected emotionally by these events. The sad thing is that the origin of the grief that is carried from the loss is almost impossible to detect in normal therapy.

This opens one great question that so many people have around the VTS:

*In the early months the foetus does not have the physical capacity to hear or see, let alone sense or remember experiences beyond the placenta, so who remembers?*

Who remembers, indeed! Jenny Wade and David Chamberlain are two among many who have published widely on verifiable adult memories of experiences in the womb.[5] These are so precise that we have to conclude that there is a witnessing medium capable of sensing and remembering during parturition. This 'witness' is present in, or in the vicinity of the foetus and the mother all through pregnancy. It seems to be related in some way to the Higher Self, or perhaps the soul.

Using this concept with our clients during therapy is the most effective way to create a healing ambience. We refer to the one who senses and remembers as their true Self, and that the loss in the womb is an arrangement made between Selves.

Let us now discuss what is it in a clients' behaviour that may indicate the presence of a VTS? We have already published much of this on the web. By adulthood the impact has usually become quite subtle and is less focussed than more recent traumas from childhood. Among many 'symptoms' the most important is that they never understand why they should be constantly plagued by feelings that have no apparent cause. They find it really hard not to know what is driving them all the time. They feel different from others, and very alone. Some of the symptoms are contradictory, and typical of what psychologists would call separation anxiety:

- *Ineffable but profound sense of loss, loneliness, abandonment*
- *Will act out against others neurotically, or against themselves masochistically*
- *Deep unarticulated fear that loss will happen again, a pervasive insecurity*
- *Hard to trust, which diminishes the ability to bond except in a neurotic way*
- *Sense that others will not support them or endlessly wanting to support others*
- *Longing that cannot be fulfilled*
- *Belief that some part of them is missing*
- *Deep shock that holds back maturity so they remain childish*
- *Needing to be physically near others, often sleeping wrapped in the other's arms*
- *Yearning for the perfect partner, often resulting in co-dependency*
- *Sense that some one, or some guardian angel is caring for them*
- *Stretching towards others so they merge easily, often with imaginary friends*
- *Being extremely sensitive to the needs of others*
- *Loose or over-strong personal boundaries,*
- *Resentful at having to suffer their own birth alone*
- *Fear of or fascination with death*
- *Understanding of death that appears innate*
- *Split, so always looking outside themselves for their identity*
- *Courageous, for they have to do it alone*
- *Avoiding public display, physical contact or being looked at*
- *Fascination in twins, watching them on TV or dreaming about them*

Some symptoms, you will notice, are relatively minor.
My wife Hilary had lost a twin, has since childhood been
very interested in death experiences, and is also fascinated
with twins. Yet these absorptions were fairly relaxed and
detached. She has been strongly influenced in her life by this
event, but not traumatised. She was lucky in this, for her case
is not typical. What sets a VTS apart from others is that even
where there has been little suffering in childhood they still
have feelings of loneliness and abandonment.

In our work we find that the first level of healing comes
once the cause is understood. Here are three typical people
who got enormous benefit from realising their history:

*Sarah* would bring all her relationships to a quick end
because, though she could not have told herself why, she
could not bear the fear they would abandon her if they got
too close.

*Mary* had anorexia that turned out to be linked to her
foetal guilt that when her twin had died. Mary decided it
was because she had 'stolen' all the food.

*Bill* had spent a lifetime searching for a twin-soul
to merge with until he discovered he had had a twin of
the opposite sex, and this helped to explain why he had
passionately longed to be a girl and had thought of becoming
a transvestite.

One of the modalities we have developed at the Crucible
Valley Centre is called energetic processing. In it we use
connected breathing in a very quiet setting to support the
client to move into the deeper spaces of the psyche. It is a
soft process, yet is able to access the most profound issues
that have become embedded in the psyche from foetal times.
Combined with sandplay, this work has brought many of
these decisions to consciousness.

Here are some typical ones, and in brackets the more
common consequences:

• I took all the nourishment and he starved [*bulimia, anorexia*]
• I was responsible [*remorse, acting out war stories, self-punishment*]
• I failed because I could not keep him with me [*self-blame*]
• I feel poisoned [*becomes vegetarian, hypochondriac*]
• I blame myself for his death [*deep distrust, self-loathing*]
• I was not worthy, so I had to remain on earth [*unworthiness*]
• I will be on a spiritual path so I can follow him [*fantasy, ungrounded*]
• Why did I live and my companion die [*guilt*]
• I won't leave him [*won't grow up, retreats under stress*]

These are all common decisions people make in response to events in growing up, and are not necessarily created through the loss of a twin. It is only in an actual clinical situation with the energetic support of the therapist that the client is able to self-examine deeply enough to work out whether the decision came from the womb.

It is important to realise that in therapy the client's view of themselves is primary. We therapists listen and respond. Were we not to be, in this sense, the passive receiver of a client's truth, the client would seldom have the energetic support needed to discover themselves. It is not easy to communicate this concept in a short article, but it lies at the core of effective transpersonal psychology. How can we be sure that we are not dealing with pure fantasy? How do we know that the self-investigation is not a delusion? There is a 'ring' to the truth, an emotional wholeness that is hard to gainsay. I will give the outcomes of these cases in their own words:

*I have spent fifty years not being able to feel my body.*
*It was something that hung off me, and not in me, if you*
*know the difference. I had already traced that feeling*
*to an operation I had when I was four to remove a*
*second bowel that was strangling my working bowel. In*
*therapy I felt into the place where that bowel had been.*
*It was a huge surprise to recognise that the extra bowel*
*had been full of a happy, joyful energy, and that when it*
*was removed, that vitality went too. I concentrated on*
*drawing it back to me and had a sensation of wiggling*
*fingers and toes, but it was coming from the second*
*bowel. It seemed that that second bowel came from my*
*dead twin. I felt so different afterwards - very different*
*about everything I touched.*

In the second case, a series of unconnected memories formed
a coherent pattern for the first time when she realised what
was driving her sense of abandonment:

*I am struggling with allowing this to be the truth. It*
*seems too incredible and yet it felt incredibly real.*
*Such huge choices being made between my foetus and*
*another. It presents an unknown which is very scary.*
*I want it and I am afraid. Yet it does resonate with who*
*I am. I have a very powerful memory of the night I was*
*taken to hospital when I was five and watching my little*
*brother in a car going in the opposite direction as he*
*went to stay with our grandparents. Watching him go -*
*losing him. The clarity and strength of the feelings - like*
*losing a part of me - again. I had the same experience*
*when my first child was born. I feared he might leave*
*me, and only when he cried did I realise how tightly I*
*was holding on to him! Endlessly holding on from fear.*

The third case is the very typical response that we are being
'acted' on by feelings and impulses over which we have
neither control nor understanding. This man had no purpose

in life, and needed others to make decisions for him. He
would often panic in large spaces and would suddenly feel he
did not know where he was going. When this happened he
was unable to retrace his steps in order to find out where he
had been.

*I have spent my life continuously drifting, while waiting*
*for someone to come back and rescue me, take me away.*
*I've always felt as though I "missed the boat." I can*
*now see that I have been manifesting this 'decision' in my*
*life. It is a pattern that keeps repeating itself. No longer*
*is there any blame on myself – or on others. It feels as*
*though the decision, now it is exposed, can be dissolved*
*and transformed.*

The most effective healing procedure, we find, has three
steps. It is to remember by accessing buried and sensitive
inter-uterine feelings, to recognise them and then to forgive
the other for leaving.

However, we find that just having knowledge of the
event is not enough to really clear the matter. It is finding the
exact and very subtle tone of the embryonic response, and
defining this exactly in words so it contains the flavour of the
moment. Where it involves a decision, the precise terms of
that 'agreement' need to be spelt out. As this is becoming
clear we need to sense the full catastrophe in the cells of the
body.

In a typical case Gail allowed her body's memory to
guide her in the physical movement she had made away from
the body of the dead twin, and as her consciousness sank into
the movement, the nature of her response to that trauma grew
and became lucid. Her adult witness could then interpret
that movement in precise words. The wording that describes
the response then becomes vitally important in the healing
process. Afterwards as we absorb the reality of what has
happened and can conceptualise the response as a decision,

then we are able to follow how it surfaced in a myriad events in life. It is then that we become free of the trauma – but we never forget.

For some people a crucial part of the healing comes in how we relate to the residual guilt, or even a shame that seems to have no source. We may have had a wonderful childhood with loving parents, yet still feel a disquiet that we blame ourselves for. The answer lies in a process of forgiveness, but it is not enough to say the words or to hold some repeated affirmation. Forgiveness needs to come from the heart – truly. Gail wrote:

*I have felt that I needed to offer something to my dead twin, but felt inadequate as there was nothing I could offer that would be great enough. I had felt this at the time, as then I lacked so much substance. I have come to recognise that offering my forgiveness was the most vital part of the process. Then an amazing sense of freedom rushed though me, and I was able – that was the magic, actually 'being able' – to forgive myself for not being conscious about all this for so long.*

Sometimes these decisions can be complex. In this example one twin intended to leave, and instead made an arrangement with the other. This is unusual, but shows the power of the psychic 'decisions' that may be made and the long-lasting distortions it leaves behind. George wrote:

*I think I am a practical man, but really I'm not. I discovered two things from regression, that I had had a twin, and that this twin was the practical one while I was essentially a dreamer. I was staggered to realise that while my twin was dying in the womb I had offered to take over the practical role just to stop him leaving. Now I know why things don't work for me: it is these contradictory drives! The dreamer in me screws up the practical, while the practical undermines my dreams.*

Consider that George had two women in his life. The first was a practical down-to-earth person, while the second was dreamy and impractical. The first longed to help people while the second needed to be helped. Another client wrote that:

*It felt archetypal – that he would sacrifice his life in order to 'kick start' my journey. My closest friend died when I was 25, and at his funeral it was said that his life's purpose had been to die for many others, in the support of their journey. It cracked me up when I heard this – it felt so true for me, personally.*

Conversely, many carry a fascination with death. The may be especially in those cases where the dead foetus remained for a time in the womb before being absorbed. Gail wrote:

*All my life I had put death on a pedestal, as all the 'special' people in my life had died. I had the belief that one must be pretty special to die. It was one of the ideas I used to beat myself up with, as I thought to myself that as something "was too special, I would never be able to match that."*

Sometimes the attachment to the womb-experience can have a baleful influence over a much wider field. Jean had run many large organisations, but always found that a considerable opposition would invariably develop against her, and she had to move on. It was often made worse because she would usually have developed a special friendship with just one person. Jean knew she had had a twin, and in a later process recognised that when her twin had died she had decided that her environment was dangerous, even toxic. She reflected this belief onto her work, and when she had found her 'twin' in her special friend would project the trauma by unconsciously turning her work environment into a dangerous place for both of them.

195

Within minutes of leaving after this discovery Jean's friend rang her, anxiously demanding they have coffee together. Such an intimate connection with a surrogate twin is far from uncommon.

Intimacy can go much further than this. Sally had lost a twin, but her daughter had not. The daughter came to us when aged twelve as she was still sleeping in mother's bed, refusing to leave home for school and starting to wear her mother's clothes. She produced an extraordinary drawing of her family, with herself within the womb-space of her mother. When Sally's twin had died thirty-five years earlier her response was to go seeking him. This lead her in later years to look for the perfect match in all her friendships, and married a man who (though not like her in personality) looked her exact double. Her terror of dying and frequent panic attacks only added to the intensity of her search, and the constant fear that the search would inevitably fail. When her daughter was born there was an instant bonding. It seemed that the natures of their two Higher Selves were in close resonance. Whatever the reason, the bonding gave Sally the sense that she had at last found her lost twin.

She described the therapy as being "enlightening, and excruciatingly wonderful", and in the days that followed her daughter moved into her own room, and began to buy very feminine clothes just for herself. The healing has continued so that now both are comfortable with themselves, and the intensity of the initial bonding has faded away. Bringing a self-aware consciousness to a precise understanding of the event brought about the healing.

What we have learned from all these clients is that there is no straightforward or simple outcome to losing a twin, but that the consequences are unique to every individual who has to search into their own womb-history to discover the truth. It is then the precise definition of this truth that sets them free.

At the end of our workshops we suggest each participant choose a card from the Rajneesh Tarot deck. We find that the advice the card gives is almost always appropriate and helpful, and emphasises the synchronicity and connectedness in all life. The card that Jean chose after a session on her twin was called "Rebirth moment to moment" and read:

*Even where your own feelings are completely justified, be open to the possibility of something beyond anything you've ever known. Jump out of the past experience into an entirely new dimension.*

## References

1. L. Sulak, M. Dodson (1986) The vanishing twin: pathologic confirmation of an ultrasonographic phenomenon, *The American Journal of Obstetrics and Gynaecology*, lxviii: 811-15.

H. Landy, L. Keith (1998) The vanishing twin: a review, *Journal of Human Reproduction* (Update) iv, 177-83.

2. Our web site is www.cruciblecentre.com

3. John James (1994) *Notes to Transformation* (available on the web, via www.johnjames.com.au)

4. Ruth Ammann (1991) *Healing and Transformation in Sandplay*, Open Court Publishing Company, Chicago,

Estelle Weinrib (2004) *Image of the Self: The Sandplay Therapy Process*, Temenos Press, Cloverdale USA

5. Jenny Wade (1998) Physically transcendent awareness: A comparison of the phenomenology of consciousness before birth and after death, *Journal of Near-Death Studies*, xvi, 249-275

David Chamberlain (1992) Are telepathy, clairvoyance and 'hearing' possible in utero? Suggestive evidence as revealed during hypnotic age-regression studies in prenatal memory, *Pre- and Peri-natal Psychology Association of North America*, vii,125-137.

# DENICE M. MOFFAT MS, DVM, ND

## THE GIFT OF A VANISHED TWIN

*"I had a twin!?" I was thinking? Here I was standing on stage in front of 250 people that I didn't even know, 400 miles away from home, having been exposed to a concept I had never heard of, and finding out something that had shaken my life permanently with no one to support me in the process.*

~~~~~

Dr. Denice Moffat is a veterinarian and Certified Traditional Naturopath through the American Naturopathic Medical Association. She has a Master's degree in Biology, a Bachelor's in Animal Science, is certified in Contact Reflex Analysis and is a Teaching Karuna Reiki Master. She has taken classes in Neuro Emotional Technique, Cranio-Sacral Work, and has taken Dr. Randy Robirds' Ener-Chi Quest Seminars. She currently focuses on human and pet health preventative medicine.

*Original, previously unpublished article.*

# 17

## THE GIFT OF A VANISHED TWIN

*Denice Moffat*

Lawrence Wright's article, *Double Mystery* published in
the New Yorker, August 7, 1995 explained that one out of
eighty or ninety live human births produces twins. With the
advent of ultrasonography it has been determined that at least
one-eighth of all natural pregnancies begin as twins. The
first ultrasound detects twins and the second one does not.
So what happens to these twins? With the use of emotional
clearing work, I often detect a vanishing twin.

### My story of how I found I had a vanishing twin

It was the summer of 1996. I was down in Southern
California taking a continuing education course for my
naturopathic degree. I had chosen Scott Walker's Neuro
Emotional Technique class. I didn't know much about the
technique and had never experienced it before, but many
people in the Contact Reflex Analysis classes I had taken had
highly recommended it, and I did need something to give me
those credits…Little did I know what was in store for me and
how my life would be changed forever.

The first day of the course went fine, but there were
huge amounts of material to assimilate and it was all new to
me. Armed with the manual that was given to us in class, I
headed back to my room to read it cover to cover to prepare
myself for the next day's lecture.

I came upon a reference page in the back of the manual
on the Vanishing Twin Syndrome. As I read the page, I
starred it, feeling an urgency to order all the recommended

articles written by Lawrence Wright. This was strange because I normally didn't purchase all the extras and I really didn't know why I was attracted to the twin articles. "Maybe it was because of the two sets of twins I had once had as friends while growing up," I thought and read on.

The next day, class continued, only they passed out another manual and we did nothing with that first manual! That unnerved me a little, but what does one do? I just went with the flow. Dr. Walker and his wife, Deb, were using people in the audience to teach their techniques. Since I had several health challenges, I raised my hand when they asked for a volunteer, but they did not choose me.

The last technique of the course was presented and they asked for a volunteer who had a long-standing problem that had not been helped with allopathic or alternative medicine. I raised my hand.

> "I have had menstrual cramps all my life, have tried various techniques—probably over 40 in my lifetime and still can't find a solution for them."

I found myself on stage being worked on by one of the best in the field. "Now we're getting somewhere." I thought. Dr. Walker worked utilizing the muscle-testing technique, using my arm as the reference muscle group. As he tested, he came to my ovaries and uterus then stopped, and hesitated. He made a three-point triangle with this thumb, index and middle finger and placed one digit lightly on each organ. Retesting with my arm made my arm weaken.

I was concentrating so on trying to see and understand what he was doing; I didn't really know the ramifications of his testing. "Oh, here's an interesting finding," he said. "You'll have to be careful how you bring this up to your clients, as it's both interesting and can cause a lot of emotions to come up—especially when you don't have a lot of time between cases." The audience laughed.

"You see how when we test each ovary and the uterus separately, how her arm stays strong for the testing? Now, by testing all three together, do you see how her arm drops?" he asked the room full of 250 doctors.

"Now...How about the concept of a vanishing twin?" He asked, as my arm  weakened for the question. "And how about the concept of male twin?" My arm stayed strong. "...And the concept of a female twin?" My arm weakened.

"So let's double-check our work," he said. "How about the concept of a vanishing twin sister?" My arm weakened. "A vanishing twin sister that died one month in utero? ...Two months in utero? ...Three months in utero? ...Four months in utero?" My arm weakened again.

"So, there's an emotional memory of a vanishing twin sister that died at four months in utero?" My arm again weakened.

*I had a twin!? I was thinking?*

Here I was standing on stage in front of 250 people that I didn't even know, 400 miles away from home, having been exposed to a concept I had never heard of, and finding out something that had shaken my life permanently with no one to support me in the process. I stood there in shock— stunned. My head was in a fog as I desperately tried to comprehend everything this man was now talking about after my mind had been filled to capacity the day before and had no more space for saturation since 10:00 a.m. this morning. I was instantly, emotionally wasted.

The class ended and I got off the stage. The attendees departed and so did I—straight for the hotel bar. Normally a light-weight drinker, I heard myself order two double Kamikaze drinks to go, and took them up to my hotel room. I drank them both!  "What's happening? ...I can't believe this…" I said over and over as all the pieces of the puzzle to my life started to fall into place.

I thought back to what my mother had told me of my conception and her pregnancy with me as bits and pieces of what I had just experienced intertwined.

Three to four months in utero is about the time the twin "checks out" and is being reabsorbed by the body. What are some causes? Some include getting hit in the stomach, car accidents, falling, emotional trauma, experiencing high fever from an illness, violent vomiting, etc.

I was my mother's first child. The oldest of five and the only daughter. She fell down a flight of stairs when I was four months in utero.

If you were born before the 60's, which I was, there were no ultrasound machines, so a twin could have easily been missed. An x-ray was only rarely taken because of the fear of unnecessarily exposing the baby to radiation.

I was born in a Catholic teaching hospital. Mom had volunteered to have interns be present during my birth. The birthing process had taken about 36 hours. I had assumed it had taken this long because of all the extra bodies being present. She had told me that the interns had checked for dilation and crowning so often that she was literally exhausted and severely dehydrated. This was her first experience with birthing and she was nervous. Fathers were not allowing in the room during the process.

Thinking back to my reproduction and endocrinology classes, I now thought about the birthing process and what would cause an extended parturition…

When you have one baby ready to come out, the placenta (the sac that contains the fetus) and the pituitary gland produce a certain amount of a hormone called oxytocin (also called pitocin). The function of oxytocin is to cause muscular contractions to push the baby out. So, if there are two babies, there is a proportionately larger amount of oxytocin. But, if one of the fetuses dies, there is not enough oxytocin to push out the extra residual placenta associated with the dead fetus. Therefore, the birthing process takes much longer.

These days, a cesarean section is performed when this type of shutdown occurs to take the stress off the fetus. Maybe mom's birthing took so long because there was not enough oxytocin being released?

In those days, even if there were an extra placenta expelled, the mother would not have known about it because the doctor usually protected the patient from information they thought would cause more stress. Did the nurses know? I've talked to midwives who said they sometimes don't tell the mother about a second placenta. One nurse even shared that she had several of them stored in her freezer for teaching purposes and that she was waiting for the right time to have a special burial for these twins tissues.

Most often the surviving twin manifests survivor's guilt for taking nutrition or causing the death somehow of the vanishing twin. Once identifying this occurrence, the patient must go through the grieving process like in any death of someone that means a great deal to them. They experience abandonment, loss, guilt, grief and anger at being separated from the twin. Sometimes the twin survivor does not care if they live or die and may occasionally have thoughts of suicide.

My childhood life was replete with all kinds of allergies, which are common for children with extended birthing times. I held stress in my chest which lead to asthma at times. Oriental medicine teaches us that the lung is the organ that holds grief. Could it be that I was causing some of this myself with survivor's guilt? I had always felt so alone in the world, always searching for "someone like me."

Twins have a special energetic bond with each other which lasts their entire lives. Because a twin leaves you in utero, this does not break that energetic bond. And if you don't feel your twin still around you, naturally you would be attracted to twin energy. I had two sets of twins as friends while I was growing up.

The surviving twin often has control issues which may be based on the premise that since they couldn't control what happened *in utero*, they are doing everything in their power to control everything they can now.

*Control and feeling out of control had always been a major issue in my life.*

Survivors don't usually like competitive sports unless they are competing against themselves. They subconsciously feel that if they compete with others, death may result. They want everyone to get along and work together.

I hated competition with a vengeance. "Why can't everyone just get along?" I'd ask. I was always the peace-keeper and connector. I worked on the competition issues after the Neuro Emotional Technique class because I found these feelings were holding me back in the business world.

*Competition kills people* is what came up. Hmm.

My mother did smoke. Studies show that smoking lowers the oxygen content of the blood, so less oxygen is available to the fetus. Smoking is also associated with low birth weights. Does that mean there is less available oxygen and nutrition for two fetuses? Did I compete with my twin sister, taking "all" the oxygen and nutrition and leaving too little for her?

"Did I kill her?" I thought in horror.

Then again, it would make sense that not every egg is perfect and not every sperm is perfect. When the imperfection is too great, problems can occur in regards to the available nutrition for one or both of the babies. When this happens, the fetus starves and is then resorbed back into the body. The remaining fetus then has enough nutrition to grow to full-term. We see this all the time in the veterinary world. Do animals have a sense of loss and suffer from Vanishing Twin Syndrome as well? This new insight led to a cascade of emotions, involving working through low self esteem and self-worth issues.

Low self-esteem is intertwined with a lack of unconditional love of the self, trust and discernment and low self-worth issues. These are the major Spiritual lessons that the twin survivor must work through before they can fully be the gift to the world that God intends. Although many other people without twins also have to work through these issues, I see these lessons every time with those who have a vanished twin.

I also had to work through the feelings of being abandoned (*why would she leave me—am I a bad person? Was there something wrong with me? If my own sister wouldn't be with me, then why would a mate?*)

Sabotaging happens when relationships start going too well. The superconscious/subconscious thinking is that whoever they get close to will be in danger and might die from their actions somehow. Because they love someone, they will push them away to protect them and to pay for what they have done to their vanishing twin.

Yes, I had sabotaged several relationships in my life. Most relationships I did develop were not healthy ones. I gave too much, expected too little and did not value my time or my life. This stifled my Spiritual growth. I didn't know any better because I could not see any other way to act. I was not ready to let go of my "stuff."

I went through a period of time while attending veterinary school, where every close friend of mine died. In my subconscious it planted a seed that whoever became close to me would die. When relationships would start to go well for me, I wondered what was going to happen to destroy the partnership—or should I be breaking it off to protect them?

Surviving Twins often work in the healing fields. Since they could not heal the situation in utero, they are intent on healing the world and saving others. There are lots of surviving twins who are massage therapists, doctors, nurses, chiropractors, nurses assistants, midwives and veterinarians.

The survivor often feels they don't deserve all the good this world has to offer. They find ways to exclude themselves from receiving good. They are very hard on themselves—harder than anyone else could be, and punish themselves for things others would just let go of and move on. They are major givers, but not very accepting takers or receivers.

Surviving Twins are motivated people. Because they find it hard to love themselves, they look for it from their external environment. "How could we have done this without you? You're the best!" is what they live for. So they expend energy on things that are not fun for them. They volunteer for projects that no one wants to do—even if they don't want to do it either, and overcome insurmountable odds to look like a hero.

Because they do such good in the world, often money follows. The problem is that vanishing twins don't seem to be able to hold onto the money because of their self-sabotaging. Survivor's guilt prevents them from using the money for their own care. They give it away or let it flow through their hands, not keeping any of it for themselves.

Feeling abandoned, left out, and excluded is another trait of a vanishing twin survivor. These are the kids who get picked last for the team, who don't make friends easily and feel like others can't relate to what they are going through. They are searching for close relationships but can't seem to find them. Often they would rather spend time with older people than kids their own age.

I had always felt like the "black sheep" of the family.
I had few friends, and fewer yet female friends. There was
never really anyone I felt that close to—someone that I could
trust totally my own age. Stranger yet, each time one of my
brothers married, I overreacted. "Oh! I finally have a sister!"
Evaluating my reaction, I'd think, *Why'd I say that?*

As with all people gifted with a Vanishing Twin I found
that Spirit moves in Divine Right Order. Along the way I
attracted clients, situations and healers into my life that were
going through the same processes so that I could see how the
Vanishing Twin Syndrome was handled in many different
ways and stages.

At one workshop a woman came up to me and told me
she could see that I was not in my body and that my body
was inhabited by a twin. She asked me if I would like to be
"reintegrated".

"Well...sure." I said hoping that my skepticism was not
showing through. What I was really thinking was, "This girl
is a nut-case weirdo, but I doubt she can hurt me and it will
make her feel useful."

Strangely enough, after that day no one has called
me "airhead," "ditz," "space cadet," "dizzy," or any of the
other words people had often used to describe my actions
and way of thinking. I also had been severely directionally
challenged before that day. Now my sense of direction
seems to be average, and I'm better with numbers than I've
ever been before the reintegration.

Often, clients and people who see my web page on
the Vanishing Twin Syndrome will write to me and tell me
their story. All are fascinating examples of how they came
to discover they have a vanishing twin. They ask me the
significance of their situation and what I think.

I think that the fact that the vanishing twin came up in
their life at this time is perfect. The body does not allow
these things to reveal themselves until we are ready to work

through the issue using this piece of information on our soul's journey and evolution. That little soul that came and left so quickly chose to be in the lives of the mother and its surviving twin. All individuals get the gift of that energetic interaction.

After we work through the shock of discovering a twin, we meet others on the same path so that we can totally and completely immerse ourselves in the experience seeing the situation from all different angles. We will meet people in various stages working through their own issues with self esteem, self-worth and unconditional love of the self so that we can see how much we've accomplished and where we need to go.

These are mentoring interactions that are best embraced to be as complete as we can in this lifetime's journey to perfection. Whatever we are going through right now is right and perfect. As with all emotional traumas, we need to be gentle with ourselves and search/ask our Higher Power to be shown the gifts that are to come from these experiences.

I have now had several years of working through all the emotional and physical aspects of this journey for me. I am a better person for it and a talented practitioner in a field I had traveled into from the world of medicine and into the world of metaphysics "kicking and screaming on the way to transformation." I realize that what my twin gave me was a special gift and that her soul journey and mine are interconnected and tied together on a bigger scale somehow.

I never did find a resolution for the menstrual cramps, but now I am approaching menopause and they have almost gone away. I will say that I have resolved many issues having to do with the cramps that I had encountered over my lifetime. I've found ways of working though and forgiving many well-meaning treatments and have come to terms with my victimhood about having cramps. I've often wondered if part of the cramps was grieving over children lost in past lives and dying during childbirth, but mostly I think they are from contraction of the uterus against the fibrous strands adhering to it from a ruptured appendix when I was 16 months of age.

I also realize that I am not alone. My twin sister is with me always, but now stands behind me in support. She does not inhabit my body any longer because I've grown and am strong enough to be in my own body and have accepted my own assignments in this lifetime. I'm no longer depressed. I love my life. My daily mantra is now, "It's all good."

# SHIRLEY A. WARD Med.Dip.Ed.

# SUICIDE AND PRE-AND PERINATAL PSYCHOTHERAPY

*The relationship between negative events from conception to birth, and suicide, are explored. From extensive experiential work with clients, based on the work of the British psychiatrist Dr Frank Lake, the author stresses that something else is going on in every death by suicide, that is not visible. Hidden factors relating to suicide have their roots in the pre- and perinatal period, from as far back as conception to the birth itself.*

~~~~~

Shirley Ward is Education Director of the Amethyst Resource for Human Development based in County Clare, Ireland. Having taught for twenty two years she now works as a pre- and perinatal psychotherapist and educator having researched foetal consciousness for over 25 years. She is an international advisor to APPPAH, (Association for Pre- and Perinatal Psychology and Health) in USA.

*A shorter, edited version of an article originally published in APPPAH Journal (USA) Volume 19, Number 2 Winter 2004. Reproduced with permission*

*Amethyst Resource for Human Development, Amethyst, Ballybroghan, Killaloe, Co Clare, Ireland*

# 15

## SUICIDE AND PRE-AND PERINATAL PSYCHOTHERAPY

*Shirley A. Ward*

### Introduction

Looking for that which is not visible is at the foundation of pre- and perinatal psychotherapy when working with those who are suffering the excruciating pain that can be at the primal roots of suicidal tendencies.

Since it was founded in 1982, the Amethyst Resource for Human Development in Ireland[1] has pioneered and researched the experiential work of over two thousand five hundred people reliving their journey from conception to birth. This has been experienced through the techniques of pre- and perinatal psychotherapy, primal integration, regression therapy, energy healing, visualisation, meditation, art work, shamanic journeying, music, gestalt and other humanistic and integrative therapies.

These methods have been used working side by side with the rapidly growing science of pre- and perinatal psychology, which is dedicated to the indepth exploration of the psychological dimension of human reproduction and pregnancy. This includes the mental and emotional development of the unborn and newborn child based also on the work of the British psychiatrist, Dr Frank Lake. Evidence has shown that stressful pregnancies, traumatic births, and as far back as disharmony and conflict at conception, may hold the key to subsequent adult behaviour, relationships, attitudes, diseases we develop and the blocks that inhibit human potential. Within all these complicated issues of humanity are those of suicide and attempted suicide. It is my belief that at any point during the conception, pregnancy or birth, where the pain of the single cell, the blastocyst, the foetus, the preborn, is beyond the point of bearing, suicidal thoughts and tendencies take their roots.

## The retrieval of pre- and perinatal memories

The retrieval of pre- and perinatal memories, from before and around birth, and including as far back as conception, can help us understand how and why we behave as we do in the world. The deep parenting, and spiritual parenting of our own self discovery of those primal times begins to heal what might have gone amiss in the conception, gestation and birth from our physical parents

That conception, gestation and birth may have been wonderful or terrible. Remembering helps the re-creation of us. It creates the deep healing of what went wrong - and the deepening realisation of what went right.

It is important to remember and experience the positive, in order to empower our whole being and to overcome negative blocks, which have hampered the development of human potential. Many answers are found in these periods of human development, the study of which is still in the infancy stage.

Since his death in 1982, the work of Dr Frank Lake has made a major impact upon the realms of pre- and perinatal psychology worldwide. He spent many years of his life exploring the realms of conception, the first, second and third trimesters of life in the womb and the effect upon later personality and behaviour.

Until recent years the common scientific practice has been to approach the earliest period of human development, from conception to birth, as a period of quiet time in the womb, where nothing happens. The belief being that Baby

lives for nine months inside Mother's womb, cosy and warm,
protected and comforted by Mother and Father. Nothing
could be further from the truth in many cases and neither is
the belief that life begins at birth and not before.

## The difficulty of verification

For those who have not experienced this work and others
who are deeply sceptical, and often misinformed, it is vitally
important, before continuing to look at the primal roots of
suicide, that the general understanding and knowledge of
how that which may be invisible to us from the very early
times may be made known to us.

The major question is so often asked how this cell
consciousness, foetal memory or birth trauma can be real.
The most convinced person is the one who has experienced
the hidden places of life, from a primal place so far back, that
it is difficult for them to comprehend. The experience has
modified symptoms of major life difficulties profoundly. In
the case of suicidal tendencies, having found them at source,
the emotions and desire to end it all have dissipated in some
clients. Once the place where the emotions originated have
been found and the client realises that these feelings do not
belong in the present day, there is great hope and often a
positive behaviour change for the future.

## Verifying cellular memory

Dr Lake[2] posed the questions of verification alongside the
question of the embryological one. In the 1970's he was
attempting to prove it was physiologically conceivable
that the cellular and primitive body-brain functions of the
organism at six to twelve weeks could cope with the complex
tasks of findings from deep experiential work.
Taking this all back to conception, Dr Lake believed that
it was possible that in the protein molecular structures of

that single cell there is a capability to react to internal and external, good and bad, pleasurable and noxious stimuli. He stated that it was obvious to anyone who had studied the singe cell amoeba, that a single cell could do so much.

## Molecules of emotion

Candace B. Pert PhD [3] after years of research discovered the opiate receptor and many other peptide receptors in the brain and body, which led to an understanding of the chemicals that travel between the mind and the body. She discovered that the brain makes its own morphine, and that emotional states are created by the release of the chemicals called endorphins, shorthand for endogenous morphines.

This pioneering research has shown how our internal chemicals, the neuropeptides and their receptors, are the actual biological underpinnings of our awareness, manifesting themselves as our emotions, beliefs and expectations, and profoundly influencing how we respond to, and experience our world.

The molecules of emotion run every part of our body. In our world of the Establishment meeting the New Paradigm the scientific answers are there for those needing them. In the pre- and perinatal areas of discovery this knowledge adds a vital understanding to Dr Lake's theories of the maternal foetal distress sydrome, and F. J. Mott [4] who named his theory "negative umbilical effect." In other words, anything that is happening to the pregnant mother, whether positive or negative, influences the foetus through the umbilical cord and the whole of the womb environment.

## Two perspectives of studying birth and intrauterine memories

Today researchers are studying birth and intra-uterine memories and movements from two perspectives. Firstly, scientific studies of the activities of the unborn and newborn baby are being documented, particularly the unborn, with the use of ultra sound scanning of the foetus in utero. So from before birth, ultrasound is revealing the hidden life of the unborn baby.

The second perspective is that of birth and womb experiences relived by adults, children and babies in regression therapies or other body related therapies and hypnosis. It is through the experiential work that the following stories are told.

## Healing suicidal feelings:

### A Case Study of a Client working between 1977 and 1980.

*This account was written by a client working with us more than 25 years ago - this is to show that the work lasts and is not just a short-term fantasy.*

On reflection I had a severe schizoid personality disorder. It caused me such great distress and pain that it was easier for me to cut off from the pain than allow myself to feel the suffering at a deep level. Consequently I lived my life at a superficial level and the pain was well hidden.

But at times when it surfaced and became intolerable I wanted to die. I first attempted suicide at the age of thirteen with an overdose of pills. At the time I had no idea why I had done this - but parental illness, my own physical pain and family financial pressures caused intolerable responsibilities that I was too young to deal with. I had thought about ending it all, many times.

My own regression work as an adult took me to the earliest places in my life when I experienced the primal pain of rejection through attempted abortion, more than once, and the most horrific forceps delivery that felt like it was severing my head from my body. I had no idea that my therapy would take me into these places and I certainly

215

had no knowledge that the human organism was capable of remembering so far back.

In regression therapy I had relived the loss of my twin sister at the point of implantation. This appeared to be the roots of the schizoid place, where throughout my life I was absolutely terrified of becoming close, or having an intimate relationship because of a deep fear of losing the other person. This became a life script of not being able to cope in close relationships.

But the feelings that used to rack through my body every time I went into new situations took me into reliving my birth situation of rejection, fear and horror of not being wanted. I could relate superficially but wanted no closeness. I always sat close to doors and windows in a room - I realised later it was a way of escape if people got too close. I often wanted help from others but spurned it. I felt I needed help but in no way would accept it and became known as a very independent individual.

But underneath the pain were intolerable feelings of rejection and annihilation - caused by the attempted abortions - which eventually led to very fast car driving, and car accidents, which thankfully involved no-one else, and did not kill me or anyone else, although unconsciously I now know the suicide attempts were there.

I am aware that therapists may be filled with empathy and compassion but be baffled why a certain individual experiences herself at the core of her being as so utterly wretched and worthless. But finding out either from mother or the client experiencing what mother's feelings were, when she realised in shocked recognition that she was pregnant has had a terrible impact on the growing foetus. That this 'new life' was a disaster which mother both feared and hated intensely, and mother's feelings transfusing 'the foetus', who often is aware of being a loathed object and not a person, are other places during pregnancy which have a devestating personality affect, all of which becomes projected onto present day life.

My own feelings of suicide were illogical but after reliving the trauma and stress of the pregnancy and birth I realised there was a real place in life from where these feelings came. This was the healing. The change of behaviour came from knowing I was not mad. It was no-one's fault. There was no-one to blame. At that time my parents did not know that anything negative that was happening in their lives was coming into me.

I no longer have suicidal feelings because they do not belong in the present. I was meant to live - not die young. But if I had not learned the primal place where these feelings had originally come from I would have died by suicide over twenty- five years ago. I understand that with this prenatal distress percolating into adult life it is no wonder these early primal events are projected and cause suicidal tendencies.

## 2003: A more recent experience of discovering where suicidal feelings originate

*At the time of writing this young woman had only recently discovered where her feelings of suicide and wanting to die, originated.*

In telling you my story, and my struggle to both live and die, it involves the struggle to survive my inheritance from both my parents. My fight has been to break the cycle, not only for my sake, but also for the sake of my children.
My mother had a history of difficult births, and I was the seventh. My mother's first delivery almost ended in her death. Her life hung in the balance for almost a week following an emergency caesarian. I was 10lbs 11ozs in weight and was delivered by forceps. In retrospect I lived my childhood in the shadow of fear. As I entered puberty, life was going to get worse. Life began to terrify me.

It was terrible. My fear intensified and I was afraid to move in case I moved the wrong way. At the age of 16, a year after taking my first drink I began to suffer from depression. I couldn't figure out what was happening to me and I decided that life was not worth living and I had my first suicide attempt - overdosing on aspirin. I was in such emotional pain and didn't know how to deal with it. My only way of killing this pain was either to get drunk or overdosing.

I married young and had two children. For seven years I spent my time at home pretending I was happy. I was far from happy and felt very trapped. I sank deeper and deeper into depression and became addicted to the antidepressants prescribed by my doctor. They blanked out what I was feeling- and the suicide attempts I experienced in my teens, resumed.

Death was when I would have it made and I decided the only way out of my marriage was to kill myself. Two weeks before Christmas I went to bed taking over a month's supply of antidepressants. It was the first time I felt hope in a long time - that death was my only hope. My suicide was unsuccessful and I woke up in intensive care two days later.

My children lived with my husband - I left and attended the day hospital for treatment but ended up for a month in a mental home. I got a part time job and joined A.A. and went into counselling. I was grieving for my lost childhood and I wanted it back. The trauma I had experienced over the years could have a two- fold effect. It could be the catalyst for creative change or the cause of self-destruction. I had done the self- destruction bit - I was now ready for the creative change.

I discovered whilst doing regression work that I spent nine months in my mother's womb being totally ignored by her. I felt my mother's reaction to her pregnancy such as ignoring me, hoping that I was a false alarm, and then

anger towards me when she realised she was pregnant. Her
reactions had a profound effect on my attitude not only
towards her, but also towards how I felt about myself.
I had nine long months to marinate in all this negativity and
shame that my mother felt towards her pregnancy. Her lack
of recognition led me to feel unwanted, rejected and shamed.
My birth scripts, which became life scripts, were reading,
'I'm not wanted', 'I'm a mistake', and 'I shouldn't be here',
'I don't belong'. During my delivery my mother refused to
help me being born, and my terror of being suffocated and
dying in the womb resulted in me having a profound sense of
anger towards her for trying to kill me.

However, how was my mother to know that her own
thoughts and feelings would have such a deep effect on
me inside the womb? I myself was brought up with the
knowledge that babies couldn't ever hear or see for weeks
after being born, never mind being able to hear and feel
inside the womb!

It was very emotional for me to learn that these maternal
attitudes and feelings could leave a permanent mark on the
unborn child's personality. I feel tremendous gratitude that
I am able to connect the fractal patterns in my life from
conception to the present time. I feel my compulsion to die
through suicide came from the trauma I felt in the womb
and the feelings I was marinated in; my mother's feelings
and mine, became all confused - 'I shouldn't be here', 'I'm a
mistake', and 'I'm going to die during this delivery.'

My way of attempting suicide through overdosing on
medication can be connected to Mam taking medication for
her migraine and blood pressure whilst pregnant with me.
I was recreating time and time again through events in my
life, my time in utero and birth trauma.

I feel certain that my mother's fear of death and dying
came from being conceived herself after her sibling died at
the age of six weeks. She would have been marinated in her

own mother's feelings of grief, and her fear of perhaps losing
her own baby.   By relating all of these fractals I am able to
free myself from the destructive patterns at work in me.
I can now differentiate what problems were mine and what
problems were my parents'.

**How the process works**

In experiential psychotherapy, regression is part of a process
of diminishing one's defences against internal reality of
pain and trauma.  The stories included show how a person
'acts out' their pre- and perinatal dynamics in gruesomely
overt ways of suicidal tendencies because the dynamics
are so hidden, repressed and overlaid with defenses that
the conscious mind has absolutely no access to, or insight
into them being part of their unconscious dynamics.  The
conscious mind is then completely able to convince itself
that these dynamics are actual and real parts of the situation
and therefore require an actual, real and extreme response.
Adzema[5] explains that this can be brought about by a total
dissociation from one's pre- and perinatal traumas - but the
trauma is internalised and self- inflicted, and in this situation
the suicide may be completed and death occurs.

When there does not exist that total and complete
dissociation of the pre- and perinatal trauma, and it is much
closer to the surface, although still not in consciousness, it is
more likely to be allowed to emerge into consciousness, be
relived, healed and then removed forever as a motivation to
end one's life.

**Questions relating to the phenomenon of suicide and pre-
- and perinatal theory**

I am aware that there are two very important questions
relating to suicide to be answered by any theory that tries
to explain the phenomenon of suicide.[6]  The first is why
a particular person wants to take their own life, as it goes

against the survival instinct. The second is the specific type
of suicide chosen by the individual.

*Why would a particular person want to take their own life?*

When working in the area of pre- and perinatal
psychotherapy and psychology, relating to suicide, we see the
patterns emerging from early experiences in a human life that
prove to be a direct transcript of death being the only way
out, and they have to do it themselves. At the time it may
only have been temporary, but it was sufficiently imprinted at
a cellular level for the person to have stored in their psyche,
memory and consciousness, that they have to end their lives
to find peace; they have to eliminate the unbearable pain; and
the pattern is that they must kill themselves. There are many
other reasons why a person wants to take their own life, but
this is the reason we have found in the deep experiential
work. If it is not possible to survive, as the odds are too
great against the organism, the only answer is to end life.

*Why is a particular type of suicide chosen by the individual?*

Grof [7] claims there seems to be a close connection between
the state of mind a depressed person is in and the type of
suicide contemplated or attempted. The thoughts may not
only be to end one's life but to do it in a particular way.
In our work the type of suicide appears to co-incide or relate
to the events experienced in early life, at a particular period
of gestation or process of gestation.

## Types of suicide appearing to coincide with events in the pre-- and perinatal period

Remembering that this total opposition and transmarginal
stress can be present right from the beginnings, in the
conception stage where lust, anger, rage, rape, drunkeness,
parental neglect, contempt and detachment may be present

221

individually, or in some cases, multiple problems, and this can create a pattern throughout life.

Some people who are suicidal have never accepted their incarnarnation into life and into a physical body. They have never wanted to be here, some at a soul level, and have only wanted to 'return from where they came'.

Difficulty in implantation, and a desperation to find a place to be, can culminate in never finding the right place to be, and the isolation drives the person to suicide, when in adult life the terrible isolation becomes overwhelming. This also links when mother finds out she is pregnant and the response is negative. The whole organism feels 'I shouldn't be here', 'It's all my fault', 'I'll end it as I'm the cause of her distress'.

The loss of a twin in utero is more common than is usually imagined, and mother may or may not be aware of this, but the remaining foetus does know. The guilt on the surviving twin is enormous and the blame is heavy. The desire may be to return where the twin has gone as the pain of separation is too great.

Suicide attempts by an overdose of drugs may be related to drugs taken by mother during the pregnancy, or linked to anaesthesia during the birth process. So much of the distress in the womb from external events, causes severe pain in the foetus. The invasion of the foetus by maternal distress, from the mother's often complex emotions is experienced by what Lake [8] called the Maternal Foetal Distress Syndrome, and Mott [9] called Negative Umbilical Affect. The suffering foetus states 'I'm in a dreadful place - I can't stand it', and so the suicidal tendencies are sown. Never so deeply as the survivors of attempted abortion, deeply aware of annihilation, rejection and therefore the risk of being 'wiped out'. This deep sense of not being wanted permeates into all areas of life and the desire to end it all is great. In regression the adult reliving the feelings of this suffering foetus, knows that its life is in danger and relives its own near-murder with quite shocking accuracy and overwhelming terror.

Elisabeth Noble [10] writes about the work of Canadian psychologist Andrew Feldmar [11] who, as well as researchers at Loyola University in Chicago, found that some adults would attempt suicide at the same time each year. This was to do with timing, and these attempts turned out to be related to the month in which the mother had tried to terminate the pregnancy. The survivors also had used a method of suicide similar to the mother's abortion attempt, instruments or chemicals.

## Birth trauma and suicide

The process of birth itself for most people may be tough, but tolerable. For others it may be devastating in its destructiveness. Cataclysmic muscular convulsions turn, in some cases, what would have been some type of peaceful haven into a crushing hell. The 'no exit' phase, before the cervix begins to open, can last for hours. The sheer horror of not being able to 'get out' instills thoughts of death being the answer to not feeling the pain. Intolerable pressures in later life may reinforce the suicidal thoughts.

Working with many of these events in adult regression in the therapy room over the last twenty-five years we believe the roots of some, if not all, types of suicide are to be found in the pre- and perinatal period. What has been produced is a lifelong imprinting of distressful feelings that have nothing to do whatever with the person's present life situations.
It is a direct transcript, extraordinary, and in specific detail of the pregnant mother's disturbance, from conception to after the birth. In the birth process, the cord round the neck could lead to hanging in later life. In one case twins were born who were not wanted. The boy was born, and nearly died at birth with the cord round the neck. At twenty-one he killed

himself by hanging. Also related to the cord, is the suicidal attempt of slashing wrists, which is a typical attack on a cut bloody cord.

## Two scientific studies

Two scientific studies were done from which statistical data on the relationship between birth trauma and suicide were published. Both sets of results found birth trauma to be a high risk factor for later suicidal behaviour. Dr Lee Salk[12] found that teenage suicide was related to birth trauma. He discovered the most significant correlation of prenatal and birth conditions in the obstetrical histories of the suicides under study. Out of ten perinatal risk factors, respiratory disorder, absence of prenatal care and chronic maternal disease had the highest prevalence in suicides when compared to two matched control groups. Each of these factors occurred independantly in 81% of the suicides studied.

In the second study on suicide and birth trauma, Dr Berti Jacobsen and Dr Marc Bygdeman[13] discovered that a painful birth may make an individual more likely to die by violent suicide in adult life. Researching in Sweden they studied the records of 645 babies suffering birth trauma in that country between 1945 and 1980. Of these, 242 died by suicide by violent means between 1978 and 1995.

They discovered that people who subsequently died by suicide were more likely to have been exposed to birth complications and were subjected to twice as many interventions at birth as their siblings, including forceps delivery. They stipulated that obstetric procedures should be chosen to minimise pain and discomfort to the infant as they might have a long term effect in adulthood. They also discovered that people who asphyxiated themselves by drowning, hanging or gas inhalations were four times more likely to have suffered oxygen deprivation at birth.

Gaining insight into the pre-- and perinatal period and using this knowledge is a powerful tool for understanding suicide and trying to prevent it. It provides individuals with an actual place from where their often intolerable and unbearable pain is coming.

## Conclusions and the future

It seems an incredible idea that people attempt suicide because something went wrong, either as far back as conception, or in utero, or with their birth process. Society is slow to recognise the importance of the primal period but the evidence of the power of imprinting from this time has increased dramatically over the last ten tears. Preconception care and the physical health of the unborn is an area where more knowledge is being given to new parents to be. Prenatal education and classes for parents go back many years - but there seems to be a gap in the care of pregnant women, probably more so in the Western world, than in the East where often the spirituality of a nation gives more energy to the developing baby.

The major sin of humanity may well be ignorance - and this is the lack of information on the area of pre- and perinatal influence on later suicide and other post traumatic stress syndromes. Behind every death by suicide are hidden factors - and the unexperienced has to be experienced to find the circuit breakers, if this is possible with a client.

Maybe the sceptics are those who have never experienced the depth of human despair and the desire to die. Being sensitive to the awareness of the pain of the client, who is in the tenderest of places, where the original pain occurred, and to believe that the client is referring to experiences that actually happened, is a responsibility we owe to them. Worldwide research is teaching us that we must expect serious consequences whenever foetal life has been subjected to maternal distress, addiction, domestic violence,[14] abortion attempts and abuse during pregnancy. The self can die in a surviving body and lead to death by suicide.

The human race has much to learn about the attitude to sex and caring relationships. There is a different dimension to be aware of, in response to the question why, in regard to suicide. The question as to why suicide occurs or is attempted need not go unanswered. It lies deep within the human psyche.

Raising children who experience the minimal amount of trauma in the pre- and perinatal period will produce happy babies and self fulfilled adults. They will live in society without the desire to end it all. I hope that more research studies will be undertaken to look at the possible links between suicide and pre- and perinatal events.

## References

1. Amethyst Resource for Human Development, Amethyst, Ballybroghan, Killaloe, Co Clare, Ireland

2. Lake, Frank.(1982) *Mutual Caring* Unpublished text. Edited and published privately by Wasdell. David. (1998) entitled *The First Trimester*. Urchin. London.

3. Pert, Candace.B. PhD. (1997) *Molecules of Emotion. Why You Feel the Way You Feel*. Scribner. New York.

4. Mott, F.J. (1965) *The Universal Design of Creation* Mark Beech.

5. Adzema, M.D. (1996) The Scenery of Healing. Commentary on De Mause's "Restaging of Fetal Trauma in War and Social Violence". *Pre- and Perinatal Journal* Vol 10 No 4 Summer 1996 pp 261-272

6. Grof, Stanislav (1985) *Beyond the Brain Death and Transcendence in Psychotherapy*. State University of New York Press.

7. Grof (1985) ibid.

8. Lake, Frank. (1981) *Tight Corners in Counselling*. London. D.L.T.

9. Mott, F.J. (1965) op.cit

10. Noble, Elizabeth. (1993) *Primal Connections: How our Experiences from Conception to Birth Influence Our Emotions, Behaviour and Health*. Simon Schuster. Fireside Books.

11. Feldmar, Andrew. (1979) *The Embryology of Consciousness. What is a normal pregnancy? The Psychological Aspects of Abortion*. D.Mall and W.Watts.eds. Washington, DC; University Publications of America.

12 Salk, Lee. (1966) Thoughts on the Concept of Imprinting and its Place in Early Human Development. *Canadian Psychiatric Association Journal* 11.

13 Bertil., & Bygdeman, Marc. (2000) *Obstetric Care and Proneness of Offspring to Suicide as Adults: A Case Control Study*. Vol 15. No 1.

14 Gilliland,Amy L., & Verny, Thomas R., (1999) The Effects of Domestic Abuse on the Unborn Child. *Pre- and Perinatal Psychology Journal* Vol 13 (3-4)

# ALTHEA HAYTON & "MARY BETH"

## FINDING THE ARTIST

*When "Mary Beth" found the wombtwin.com web site
she was very down on herself, seeking someone she could
talk with and relate to. She wasn't sure who she was, as a
twin or as a singleton, yet she knew she was not of a single
conception. Her twin brother Leslie died a cot death aged 3
months. She was trying to find some meaning and purpose
in her life and some sense of success and direction. In six
weeks of intensive work by email, we were able to discover a
tiny and mysterious part of herself, a shy artist, who had
in some sense always been there but had not
been properly acknowledged.*

~~~~~

"Mary Beth" is a poet, artist and healer and lives
in Toronto, Canada.

*An original article created from a series of emails
arising from the wombtwin.com website.
Email material made anonymous and used with permission.*

# 19

## FINDING THE ARTIST

*Althea Hayton and "Mary Beth"*

*"Mary Beth" came into my life as a chance visitor to the wombtwin.com site. She was one of many that week.*

**May 3ʳᵈ** I have only just read your web site "wombtwin" and have found some answers for myself. Thank you. I lost my twin brother, Leslie Glen when we were 3 months old and although I knew him in this life it still doesn't make things easier. I have returned many times to the womb, which I shared with my twin.

If we had not been twins and deeply connected with each other, we probably would not have survived the pregnancy, as my mother and family did not want another pregnancy or any more children. There were three already in the family. In her moments of truly wishing she were not pregnant, Leslie Glen and I embraced each other and were able to withstand her desire because of our loving bond with each other. Womb life, feelings and impressions definitely do exist and influence our daily life.

*In reply I said that to be healed she would have to be able to live without Leslie Glen and set herself free of survivor guilt.*

**May 8ᵗʰ** As a twin, I feel guilty for staying here and not going with Leslie Glen when he died. My sense of his death was that he had moved to a different space, like would happen in the womb, and then there was an awareness that this wasn't quite the same (I can't quite explain that) and it was to late for him to return to his body. As much as I wanted to go with him there was a force keeping me here. We both truly wanted to be together but it seems not both physically together. I am not truly happy with this relationship, but that is what we have.

At times, his absence seems enormous and it is at these times I feel that I wished I knew him better. Then there are other times when there seems to be a flow between us, as if we are in our own space yet in each other's space at the same time. I honestly wish I could know him better so I could give him credit for what is his, but I don't know him and never will. As the subject of being a twin was totally taboo, I was unable to discuss any of this with parents or siblings.

In my late teens I did try to find out more about what happened etc. The barrage of emotions that came from my sister and brother was hard to deal with and my mother just wouldn't say anything. My parents are both dead now and I have walked away from my siblings.

I am so glad you are there for me to talk with, although I do journal and dream. Having someone else who has also lost their twin early in life makes a great difference. I also paint and I know Leslie Glen in my muse.

*I felt a deep sense of rapport with this person, and intuitively seemed to "see" the images she was presenting to me.*

**9th May** I was caught in the tug of war between Leslie Glen and myself when he died. His wish that I come with him; my wish to go with him. It wasn't possible for me to join him or for him to return. Then from somewhere, deeper than this battle, came a wondering about who or what was the force(s) that put this struggle together.

Upon asking that question, I was aware of a force that really didn't care and was unaware of the struggle. Once there was awareness of the struggle, I (we) became free of that force. It felt more like that force let go. I felt a sense of relief and a falling apart of the tension but I was also aware of a sense of betrayal.

There is a part of me somewhere between the age of 0 to about 3 years old, that was and is very close to my twin brother. This part of me is very stubborn, determined and very suspicious of the rest of me and felt betrayed when I somehow learned to act like a non-twin to fit in with the rest of the family. It has only been within the last 2-3 years that I have finally managed to gain the friendship and trust of this irascible younger part of myself, as she now realizes that what I did was for the survival of us both.

Once I had become free of the struggle at the time of Leslie Glen's death, I then was able (I guess) to connect better with the younger part of me. It is possible that somehow that has also freed Leslie Glen to go Home.

This whole thing is also surrounded with death because, when I was 12 years old I died on the operating table. Because of Leslie Glen's death and of my death, numbness often happens in my life and I have relived (within the last 2 years) the dying on the operating table. The only reason I can figure out for reliving this, is to make me aware of my connection with Leslie Glen. After dying, that was the only awareness I had. It is as if he were reminding me I was still a twin and couldn't die yet.

Then, I was aware of a thick transparent liquid in me and surrounding me. It felt nice and it felt cleansing but I'm not sure what the clear liquid means, except that possibly I am seeing through things a bit better rather than hitting my head against a brick wall (opaque).

*The "amber liquid" and the "opaque brick wall" sounded like the amniotic fluid which is amber coloured and the opaque amniotic sac that separates twins who are diamniotic (ie. they each have separate sacs.) I have learned that these womb images can be very specific.*

**May 14th** In the next dream I found myself at about 3 years old wondering how to behave so I wouldn't always be doing the wrong thing and being punished. I decided to observe my brothers and sister and see what they did that was all right, and so I began mimicking them. What they did made no sense to me but they didn't get spanked. As I was observing, I became more withdrawn into myself and became the stubborn, irascible part of myself. Finally, I gained the friendship and trust of that part of me. When I first met her about 20 years ago, she had introduced herself as the "Orphan" and that is all she would say. I had become the Orphan, so I could finally understand why she called herself that.

Then I went back in time, in this dream, as the Orphan, to where I was a twin. I felt again that real feeling of being a twin. It was as if I had fallen into my place again. I was happy and whole. Then came Leslie Glen's death, which happened in the wee small hours of the morning. He was beside me. Late in the morning as the family woke up, his death was discovered. The noise, turmoil and jarring feelings that filled the room lodged themselves on me but, this time, in the dream, the Orphan was with me. I came through that scene with her and now have a sense of my own integrity within the twinship !!!!!!

It is interesting that all of this is happening now because on March 3rd this year I went to the emergency hospital and was there for 11 hours, with what was diagnosed as an asthma attack. I know I almost died and during that time I made some serious decisions, but not all on a conscious level. I now know I have emphysema and I wonder if on some level I was re-experiencing Leslie Glen's death. From what I know he died a crib death. I am finally feeling grounded and I am learning it is okay to be a twin and to be who I am.

*In reply I reminded her that the good air was hers, as her inheritance as the sole survivor.*

**15th May** This morning as I was waking up I became aware that I was climbing a ladder that went straight up, inside a well that was all earth. I had been climbing for quite a while and it was all dark. I was about ready to give up but I kept going and gradually I became aware of daylight. I kept climbing up until I was level with the grass and from the grass, the well shape continued, only transparent like in the other dream. I somehow knew that if I kept climbing I would go higher than the transparent walls, and that was what I was supposed to do. I kept climbing. I also woke up with an interest in painting again. Yes, it is time to live.

*I suggested a "letting go" ritual. Three hours later the same day, another email came. Clearly, Mary Beth was very engaged in this healing process.*

**15th May** I do hear you and will heed your advice. He must go!!! I thought about writing to Leslie and that might work, but painting is best. I may do a letter but the struggle is in painting, so that is best. I have attached a painting that I finished this morning. It spans the time from Jan 1st to today.

*Her picture showed an opaque field of webbed images, and behind the picture was a pool of pale blue. It seemed to be about entanglement, with multiple shreds, gradually clearing. I said that releasing a helium balloon for Leslie may help.*

**15th May** Yes, a balloon release and a long hand-written letter will help. I know he is dead and I know he is gone but something is unresolved. At this point in time, I think this is my own self-image and confidence that I can make it on my own. This morning I had an almost overwhelming sense of being homesick. I was able, during the day to track down the source of this feeling and with this came an incredible sense of love, as a twin and also as part of the Orphan. Within the Orphan, I found myself as a baby, just able to sit up on my own. This self, as a baby, was feeling very homesick for her twin brother and didn't feel at home with life without him. For her, her natural state was to be with him. I stayed with this part of me for most of the day, as best I could, and reassured her and comforted her.

I then became aware that this is the Artist in me. Now this is exciting. I also became aware that I was talking to the very, very shy part of myself who I had always been aware of but that was all. I had never before been able to get to know this shy Artist, who is now looking forward to doing some more paintings. I'll be doing the balloon release on Wednesday and probably start a new painting that day.

*I suggested that the shy Artist was that powerful, gifted side of her that survivor guilt had never allowed her to fully acknowledge. I wondered if the ritual ought to contain something male, such as blue, in memory of Leslie.*

**17th May** I passed by a place that sells balloons just tonight so I bought one and have just released it. Yes, it was pale blue with a blue ribbon. I am sure Leslie Glen is probably feeling much better now that I have found the Artist and the part of me that so longed for him. I am looking forward to doing the new paintings. The shy Artist is very powerful and really does have something to say.

*I became aware of the desperate intensity of the work we had been doing together and I suggested some time to rest.*

**17th May** I am aware of the desperation and many other things - I am also aware of something else. I am tired and do need to rest and listen. If you had not mentioned it, I would have thought I was being lazy, but "resting" is different.

*As she rested, she began to dream again with the strong imagery and story line that was characteristic of her dreams.*

**18th May** Had some interesting dreams last night. My

interest was to find the 6 month old part of me and to just
be sure I was still in touch. Then what I saw and felt was
Leslie Glen beside me and myself dead during the operation.
The numbness my body felt at both times was the same and
my body didn't understand any difference. Then gradually
I felt my body becoming alive and in this aliveness, the
Six-Month-Old appeared and gradually the confusion about
dying began to get straightened out.

In another dream, I was walking up the stairs to an old
home with the Six-Month-Old, who could now walk. We
were about 1 inch tall and the house was enormous. The
front door was a reddish wood, weather worn and simply
carved, with a rectangular and circular design. As we
approached, two figures, one from each door, like ghosts,
stepped out from the door and disappeared.

*This dream was so visual it could be painted, and I suggested
that perhaps the story could be completed that way.
I wondered, who was Beth? There was clearly something
more to find. I wondered about more twinning, and that was
why there was "something else." It is possible for a twin to
also be an identical twin and for one's "other half" to be lost
very early.*

**19th May** I've come to the conclusion that anything is
possible. I have for quite a while been debating about
painting doorways or chairs or both. Now this dream, and
your thinking of my painting it, has helped. I will begin
a painting one of these days. It really does help to write
to someone else and get some feedback, to know there are
others as crazy as myself who understand that it is important
to track these things down.

Who is Beth? I do not yet know, but am getting closer
to finding out. The shy one is not Beth, but she relates to
Beth. Yes, there may be identical twins here!!! My spirit
is a healing spirit and I have been aware since a child that I

can help people to feel better. I have for years done absent healing and laying on of hands healing, but right now it is for the healer to heal herself. The paintings that will come out of an improved state of health will hopefully benefit many.

*Her words were characteristic of what I have come to call "multiple wombtwin survivors." It was all there: the extra name that didn't quite belong; that sense of love being in the space between people; the wish to benefit and heal the others around her. I had a sense of three paintings telling a story as a whole. This idea had an instant and profound effect on her.*

**19th May** Let me sit with this for a bit. There is something (someone) inside me jumping up and down going crazy with happiness!! It is all believable. I also want to find some photographs of paintings I did a few years ago and there is a tiny girl in them and I knew it wasn't me but couldn't figure out who it was.

*Mary then completed the wombtwin.com questionnaire form and death was clearly a major preoccupation. The whole tenor of her answers spoke of a kind of spiritual malaise. The root of her difficulties seemed to be how far she was prepared to embrace life. In the complexity of her womb story there was a muddle. She could be trying to keep her other womb fellows alive in her memory, for she was the sole survivor and everyone else was dead. Her next email included a lovely picture of gently interweaving strands in purple, blue and pink.*

**1st June** I finished this on Monday and am a bit excited, as there is a new Something happening while I was painting. I like the feel of it and am encouraged to explore a new painting.

*The next email at last provided some tangible evidence of "Lilly," her identical twin, in her mother's own notes about the birth.*

**4ᵗʰ June**  When I was around 18 years old, I found amongst the books in my desk, a small book I had never seen before - my mother's notes about our birth.  There were three birth times: "(10.20 - 23 or 45?) (Boy?) (Girl + Boy)."  The doctors would not discuss the third birth.  The sense that I had an identical twin sister in the womb does truly resonate with me.

The other night I dreamed of a triptych painting that I will do a sketch of and let it grow from there.  I guess it is meant to be painted, as I now consciously recognize I am a multiple.  Because my twinship was a taboo subject, I felt it was wrong to be a twin and was not really aware of being a multiple.

I recognize Lilly, who has always been with me, but I took her for granted too often.  She came up in my journaling and I called her my Twinship Angel because I didn't know what else to call her.  The description of how she works with Leslie Glen and myself is as a "womb mate."  It is time for her to come forth in her own way, with Leslie and I, and maybe I can gain some clarity.

*Two weeks later it was clear that work on the triptych had begun and, despite the initial struggles, this was going to be a very special, healing time for her.*

**20ᵗʰ June**  I painted both sides of the triptych this morning after a week of trying to talk myself out of doing the paintings.  They are only sketches.  It is evening now and I still feel light and flexible.  The weight I've been carrying is gone and I feel like I own my body.  It was like letting go of one big bundle that was all linked together.

Now I can really consider my art career.  Thank you for walking with me.

# ELOÏSE DE HAUTECLOCQUE

## FROM DISCOVERY TO LETTING GO: MY HEALING JOURNEY

*When I discovered my twinship it made such sense and I felt such relief that my suicidal depression since about age 13 had some kind of reason behind it; I'd spent years wanting to kill myself without ever really knowing why!*

~~~~~

Eloïse is an artist and photographer living in Sydney, Australia. Originally she worked out that her twin brother must have died in the womb in the first trimester, but later on it became clear that there was more to the story.

*An original, previously unpublished article.*

*© Eloïse de Hauteclocque 2006*

# 20

## FROM DISCOVERY TO LETTING GO: MY HEALING JOURNEY

### *Eloïse de Hauteclocque*

I fit a fairly typical description of a surviving twin. I've always felt different to others and once I'd discovered my twinship I also realised that there were many clues along the way that in retrospect made such sense.

Since about 13, when I went through puberty, I started attacking my face, picking at the skin and wanting to destroy my face. Perhaps I was trying to avoid having to look at myself and to be reminded on the most subtle subliminal level, all those years, of my twin who didn't make it... I am an attractive woman and know I have caused many loved ones much grief too as they have for years tried to understand why I would want to destroy my face.

One of my on-going struggles has surfaced each month around my menstruation - I become particularly aggressive towards myself. Very self-destructive. Of course there have been many issues come up around accepting my womanhood. I am making huge progress to fully accept this side of myself, and the aggression has softened almost completely now. There are still other related physical signs that I'm working on as I resolve these physical manifestations of being a woman again in this life and an identical wombtwin survivor. There have been two stages to my healing journey: firstly when I discovered my missing brother and secondly when at last I began to recognise my identical twin sister.

239

**Finding Abélard**

I discovered I had a wombtwin five years ago, at about
29 years of age, when I started seeing a kinesiologist who
practised NET (Neuro Emotional Technique). It's hard to
explain NET in a few words, but I will try. It's a type of
kinesiology (muscle-testing technique), where you find
emotional blockages in the body and release them with a
small spinal adjustment.

You locate the block (where the energy is not flowing
easily) in the spine (nervous system) by touching points
on the body called "trigger points". These points help the
chiropractor to find which part of the body the block is in.

Then you find the emotion because each part of the
body relates to different emotions (example: liver = anger,
frustration; kidneys = fear, dread, bad memory).

You identify this emotional block in the present moment
and then you ask the body when was the first time you felt
this emotion as a negative experience. The spinal adjustment
helps to create some space where the energy is blocked and
cannot flow.

This makes me wonder about my chronic pain in my
sacral region. I know it's related to my lifelong scoliosis, the
beginning of which I've traced back to my twin's death, with
help of kinesiology, but there's more to this pain, I'm sure.

Over the years of doing yoga and other exercise
forms I've noticed blocks in my body, and particularly the
imbalance between left and right sides. I see and feel the
differences between the two sides so vividly at times and I'm
working on trying to even things up a bit because I'm pretty
much constantly in pain. My initial chiropractor commented
on how twisted my spine is, particularly down in the lumbar
region where my scoliosis is, and so I get pain in left side
upper body and right side lower body. I feel twisted. I have
since seen a medical intuitive woman who pointed out that
the real tightness is in my left hip, not the right where I feel

the pain. More recently I have noticed a tension I hold in my left leg, and even other parts of my left side, and this ties in with the wisdom that has come through about my left hip being the tighter one.

When I discovered my twinship, it was a time in my life where I felt very suicidal (which I had been on and off since about 13) after another experience of unrequited love and a close friend gave me the name of this well-known chiropractor. I finally plucked up the courage to call and make an appointment and thus I learned I started life as a twin but my twin died early in the pregnancy.

As soon as I made this discovery I was overcome with emotion and also immense relief, like finally I understood something so fundamental to who I am, why I had always felt so lonely, why I had felt different somehow to people around me. It just clicked with me and opened up a huge well of emotions ranging from anger, resentment, sadness, grief, relief. The pieces of the jigsaw suddenly started to fit together - it explained so much to me about what I'd felt all my life.

At first I thought my twin was male, because I had such a strong sense of my maleness or a feeling almost of a male presence inside me.

I was born before ultrasounds and my mother had no idea I lost a twin brother – when I told her of the discovery, she was a bit skeptical at first, which I found so hurtful. This was a discovery that was so important to me about who I am - fundamental to that, and to have my mother, who carried us both and lost one of us, not believe me was horrible.

She's coming round now, after some time... I don't know how she really feels about my twinship but she is a good listener and supports me through what I'm going through. I guess it's hard for her to be confronted with the news that she lost another baby - she miscarried before me and my twin brother. And she has never been able to grieve

Abélard, because she was unaware of him either. When I made the discovery of my twin I started to notice things that had pointed to this all along but I had just never made the connection.

My first love was with a woman who is a fraternal twin, and our relationship felt so natural to me. It wasn't an issue that we were both female, but I kept this relationship hidden, until it ended, from family and friends, because I was so frightened of being rejected by them. I told my mum when we had broken up because she asked if something was wrong, having noticed I was so down. Of course she had guessed (you can't hide things from mothers!)

I had also bonded very intensely with a girl at my school and we became inseparable friends all through school, from 10-18 years of age. She had younger twin siblings, a boy and girl, and I became closer to her younger sister who again is a fraternal twin, before I found out about my twin. We had so much in common.

I also realized I had been fascinated by pairs of identical twins at my school – one pair in my class and one in the year below. I used to play spot the differences between them privately to myself and would spend ages looking at them. I only realized all this more recently.

I had always felt so alone, different and depressed for no apparent reason, and at times I am still overwhelmed by those feelings, but discovering my twin brother's existence through NET therapy made such sense to me.

I recently had a close friend, born on the same day as me but five years earlier, share an evening with me and my family. He observed that I was so different to my family. I've always felt very close to my family (parents particularly) but aware of how I have consistently challenged them rather subtly. But my friend said to me afterwards he could see how I didn't really fit with my family, and that was so interesting. I feel we understand each other almost as twins would, and so it was an astute observation.

I believe wombtwin survivors often attract like types to ourselves, almost as if these other people provide mirrors for us. For instance I am quite sure that about four of my closest friends are also surviving twins. When I tell them of my experiences, none of them really relate what I'm talking about to themselves, but I just have a really strong instinct about it. They are all such creative loners or have major problems with relationships. If I could get them all to do an NET test to see if there was any truth for them in the idea of their being a surviving twin, I'd be fascinated to know which ones would test positive to having had a twin in utero.

All the clues were there and it was the magic missing puzzle piece, so when I discovered Abélard, I was both relieved and emotionally devastated that I had to grieve now, so long after our time in the womb.

My family doesn't really believe I had a twin brother and yet my body knows it so well!!! It made such sense and I felt such relief that my suicidal depression since about age 13 had some kind of reason behind it; I'd spent years wanting to kill myself without ever really knowing why!

At first I was often wishing that I could feel my twin brother's presence more clearly. Sometimes I felt that my cat was an incarnation of him. I've had a few dreams about my twin, only one where I saw his face. In that one we were about 2 years old or I saw him at about 2 and he was smiling up at me and looked like me but more boyish. I remember being so excited when I woke because I had seen him - I knew he had visited me. I've had others that were obviously about him but I didn't see his face.

In another dream I remember we were walking arm in arm in somewhere like Nazi Germany (I had seen this old army officer chasing us) and we were hanging out as if we could have been lovers but I knew we were just twin brother and sister. Suddenly I felt him freeze beside me and I looked behind us to see that he'd been stabbed in the kidney region and I felt all the life go out of him. It was so awful - I had this dread because I knew that it would happen almost. In that dream we were older, like in our late teens or early twenties.

## Finding Amélie

I asked a different chiropractor to check with my body what sex my twin was and I tested as having an "identical male". This confused me even more because I thought that it wasn't possible to be identical but of different sexes. I've since read that it is possible but is extremely rare. When I felt ready to let go of my twin, through ritual work, I mentioned this a bit later to another woman I see and we tested again using kinesiology. So I tested again and this time it emerged that my mother had lost a brother by miscarriage before my twin and I were conceived.

My psychologist had come across this before and referred to it as a "haunted womb". My brother's presence was very strong and he had attached to me in spirit because he needed to feel a belonging. As we worked in that session to let him go, I felt his presence leave my body quite distinctly. And then we confirmed that I had once had an identical twin.

I called my older brother Abélard (like the famous Abélard and Héloise of France), and my twin Amélie. I'd loved the French film *Amélie*, identifying with her character in many respects, and had also dreamt of an Amelia around that time. Amélie left at about 3 ½ - 4 months according to many kinesiology sessions. I think she may have completely vanished at about 4 months, but there were some sessions where I sensed a definite change at 3 1/2 months. My mum experienced bleeding at around that time so I assume that Amélie was miscarried. I tend to believe now, after much therapy, that our souls made the decision together to take our separate paths. It looks like this issue of recognising ourselves as twins is a big one for all wombtwin survivors. Most of us can't even 'prove' our twinship physically but we still identify as twins because of our strong psychic, emotional, spiritual link with our vanished twins.

## Letting go

Before I 'confirmed' my identical female twin, (I write in inverted commas because it was my body confirming the memory of that energy in kinesiology, I guess), I felt so torn also between my feminine and masculine energies. I remember being so confused by these two extremes in myself, and they were profound energy impulses. I really did feel my Abélard's energy leave my body when I identified his existence as an energy in my mother's womb before Amélie and I came into her. I decided to hold a funeral ritual by myself for both Abélard and Amélie.

After having had sunny days for the past weeks, the day was overcast and I soon saw that this was a blessing for my ritual.

I decided to buy some helium balloons and write a letter to Amélie, and also do one for Abélard and send them off into the sky. So I took my balloons off on the bus, to the sweetest comment from the bus driver "you're making the bus lighter", and looks from people on the street through the window - one guy mouthed the word 'balloons' and had such a lovely childlike look of pleasure on his face as he looked at me crowded into my seat with them. I knew I'd chosen the right symbol for me, because I feel like that too.

I had been teary that morning and felt nervous but sure, travelling on the bus to Bronte beach in Sydney, where I used to live a few years ago - really beautiful beach spot. There's a big old cemetery above the beach perched on the cliffs overlooking the sea and I chose a spot near the cemetery with a wonderful view out to sea. I walked through the cemetery

full of departed souls and knew that Amélie and Abélard
would like this place to be sent off.

You can hear the sea below and I had the company of
birds - a kookaburra (lovely Australian kingfisher type of
bird who generally sings his song before the rain), little
wrens, a magpie and others. It was relatively private in the
middle of the day on the little hill overlooking the sea - just
a few tourists doing the walk between beaches but no one
bothered me.

So I found my spot, lit a little stick of incense and wrote
my letter, first to Abélard on a blue balloon, then I wrote to
Amélie on one of the cerise balloons and the other one was
to accompany her as a symbol of my connection to her on the
spiritual plane. I had a cry as I wrote the letters and then lay
down and cut the strings from the weights that had kept them
from flying off.

I let Abélard go first and then Amélie - the two cerise
balloons. I realised how perfect it was to have this overcast
day because the sky was a clear white to watch the balloons
against as they floated away in the wind. It was beautiful to
watch and I kept my eyes on them until I could see them no
more through my tears and their distance. The lovely thing
was, Abélard 's balloon went in one direction and the two
balloons for Amélie and me went off in a different one and
they stayed together or near each other as far as I saw them.
That was lovely.

I lay on the grass for a while weeping and watching
the sky with birds and planes passing over and when I felt
strong enough I walked down the hill to the beach and had a
very refreshing little dip in the natural rock pool beside the
beach. It was cold (it was still winter here) but the day was
warm enough and it felt like the right thing to do - to bring
me back into my body. I lay on the beach for quite a while
listening to music that I'd compiled for the day and cried and
felt comforted by watching little children play with seagulls

and tourists taking photos. It was a beautiful day for it. Eventually I had some lunch, caught my bus back home and felt quite tired but calm.

**Healing**

I now see my older brother and twin sister as guides to help me empathise with both energies which are in all of us after all. I'm beginning to make peace with my essentially feminine energy and yet rejoice in the fact that I can call on the masculine in me when I need to.

I'm still learning how to trust myself to get close to another intimately. The only relationship I've had was with an older woman who is a fraternal twin, and that was way back when I was 17-21. Since then I've had intense encounters with men that never last - and I'm aware that much of that is fear that comes up in me so that I find a way to push them away. I am learning to trust that being close to someone doesn't mean death and loss... it's so hard! But I'm feeling so much more positive that it can happen, thanks to 5 years of regular treatment with chiros and a wonderful psychologist. It takes time and patience to build confidence after a loss that shaped us like the loss of our other halves.

I was diagnosed with ADD (Attention Deficit Disorder) at 33 years old, and it seems common, especially among creative people - I know many fellow artists who I would guess are ADD. Food is crucial also – personally I have found sugar to be very destructive in my diet and have eliminated it.

It is hard when no one around you really recognises you as a twin, especially family, however I am hoping if I work on my own acceptance/integration of my twinship then I won't need others' validation or acceptance of it so much. I can just let it be within me and access the richness of my twinship for myself within my life and life's work - that's what I hope for, for myself.

247

This process I am finding to be profoundly helpful in bringing about a big shift in my energy. I still feel I have work to do to "integrate" as me, but that was the beginning step of some deep work which I am continuing today.

I have to say I definitely used to feel a lot more fragmented than I do now. I used to feel such a sense of male-female energies in me, often in conflict, and yet now I feel the differences a little less.

An area of my life where I do still feel fragmented though is my career/talents. I still feel torn about which ones to focus on and somehow have a vague feeling at times that there are different "Mes" and that each talent belongs to a different "Me." I know though, rationally, that these talents are all a part of the one Me, Eloïse, and that it's OK to have many interests.

It's just a matter of letting the creative energy flow, rather than blocking it because I don't know which me it comes from. I am working towards that for now - I need to focus, and see one project through into completion.

The journey is fascinating and frustrating and liberating all at once. Last year I reached a point in my healing journey where I felt the call to help others, and so enrolled to study Transpersonal Counselling. It's been quite an adventure of self-discovery and very rich.

My true talents are creative – I have been creative since I was a small child. I particularly love photography and fashion design, both of which I have studied, but as yet I have not made them my living. I am typical of many wombtwin survivors in that respect of never quite realising all this enormous potential in me. I'm still working on that and know that I will find a way out of this stagnancy to blossom into the wondrous, creative being that I am. I'd like to find a way to bring all my talents together to help others heal - that seems like a lovely goal to work towards right now! That pain that we all know too well of the loneliness, and anguish of not knowing why we feel like this – it still brings a tear to my eye. One day recently I had such a strong image of how perfectly Amélie and I fitted together in the womb of my mother. That image made me cry and cry with longing.

I'm sure wombtwin survivors are lucky to have made this discovery about ourselves, much as it can seem like a curse at times to know a bit more... But if we find the strength in ourselves to face it, surely we'll come out of it ready for anything, and we'll attract into our lives what we really need.

I guess healing ourselves may really take a whole lifetime, who knows, but I'm hoping we get to a point where I feel empowered to achieve what I hope for, like a loving, intimate relationship with someone and success as an artist, and having a child when I find the person who feels right for me. On the whole I feel much more balanced than I have ever felt, thanks to a lot of healing work which is ongoing of course, and maybe there will always be a kind of emptiness deep inside my soul - that perhaps no one will ever fill like my twin did - but I am on my way to making a deep connection with another.

I know some pretty wise older souls who have been healing for years and say that it does become easier. It's when we let go of fears and surrender to the present that things will fall into place as they are meant to for us. The hard part is letting go of the fears and forgiving myself for all the pain I've felt. I am feeling generally so much stronger and sure of myself and I have to admit that I really feel I have let go of Amélie. I don't think about her nearly as much as I used to and when I do there isn't a feeling of pain anymore. I feel more present and happy to be here on Earth now. Wombtwin survivors have some inherent inner strength from being the survivor - and it's our job to discover it and use it to benefit everyone.

# APPENDIX A:

## SUPPORT AND INFORMATION

### FOR SURVIVING TWINS

**Wombtwin Survivors**
P.O. Box 396, St Albans, Herts, AL3 6NE, UK
www.wombtwin.com

*Information, help and healing for surviving twins whose twin died in pregnancy or at birth.*

**Lone Twin Network**
P.O. Box 5653, Birmingham, B29 7JY, UK

*Offers a network of contacts and support to anyone whose twin has died, at whatever stage of life.*

**Twinless Twins Support Group International**
P.O. Box 980481, Ypsilanti, Missouri, 48198-0481 USA
www.twinlesstwins.org

*Serving in support of twins (and all multiple births) who suffer from the loss of companionship of their twin through death or estrangement.*

**Multiple Birth Association Bereavement Support Group**
P.O. Box 105, Coogee, NSW 2034, Australia
www.amba.org.au

*Provides a means of communication in Australia for bereaved multiple birth families and surviving multiples.*

**Twin and Multiple Birth Loss NZ (Inc.)**
P.O. Box 51-984, Pakurange, Auckland, New Zealand
www.twinloss.org.nz

*For anyone at any age in New Zealand with an interest in multiple birth loss. Some adult survivor support.*

# FOR PARENTS AND PROFESSIONALS

## Center for Loss in Multiple Birth (CLIMB, Inc.)
P.O. Box 91377, Anchorage, Alaska 99509, USA
www.climb-support.org

*Serving Canada, US, Australia, New Zealand and beyond, providing parent-to-parent support for those who have experienced the death of one or both twins or multiples at any time from conception through birth, infancy and early childhood.*

## Twins and Multiple Births Association Bereavement Support Group.
2, The Willows, Gardner Road, Guildford, GU1 4PG, UK
www.tamba-bsg.org.uk

*Established 1982 in response to requests from parents who had lost a twin. Leaflets and parent to parent support group run by bereaved parents.*

## Center for the Study of Multiple Birth
333 East Superior Street, Suite 464, Chicago, IL 60611, USA
www.multiplebirth.com

*The Purpose of the CSMB is to stimulate and foster medical and social research in the area of multiple birth, and to help parents with the special problems they and their offspring may encounter.*

## The Multiple Births Foundation (MBF)
Queen Charlotte's & Chelsea Hospital, Level 4,
Hammersmith House, DuCane Road, London W12 0HS, UK
www.multiplebirths.org.uk

*Aims to improve the care and support of multiple birth families through the education of all relevant professionals.*

# FOR RESEARCHERS INTO PREBIRTH PSYCHOLOGY

**Assoc. for Pre- & Perinatal Psychology & Health**
P.O. Box 1398, Forestville, CA 95436, USA
www.birthpsychology.com

*Works to enhance the pregnancy experience and prevent birth trauma, and offer training in methods for healing the psychological wounds of pregnancy and birth. Publishers of the Journal of Prenatal and Perinatal Psychology and Health.*

**International Society of Prenatal and Perinatal Psychology and Medicine (ISPPM)**
Secretary, Friedhofweg 8, D - 69118 Heidelberg, Germany
www.isppm.de

*Devoted to the initial phase of human development - prenatal and perinatal life. ISPPM considers this earliest stage of life as the first ecological position of the human being and the womb as its first ecological environment.*

**Santa Barbara Graduate Institute**
525 E.Micheltorena St. 205, Santa Barbara, CA 93103, USA
www.sbgi.edu

*Runs a special Prenatal and Perinatal Psychology Programme, based in the belief that conception, life in the womb, birth and bonding, and the beginning experiences as an infant in the family shape our sense of self and our lives at all levels of our being-physical, emotional, mental, social, and spiritual.*

# APPENDIX B:

## INDICATORS OF A LOST TWIN

Recent research reveals that a variety of indicators do exist that a particular pregnancy that resulted in a singleton birth may have begun as twins, or which began as a multiple conception but resulted in the birth of a twin pair.

**Twins in the family**
Fraternal twinning is strongly inherited and possibly identical twinning also. Not all twins come to birth.

**Drugs to stimulate ovulation**
Clomid, oestrogen and other drugs taken to stimulate ovulation can result in a multiple pregnancy, even in a family where twins were previously unknown.

**Extra large around the waist in first trimester**
The first sign of twins can be a rapid increase in girth at the very start of pregancy, and some people begin to wonder if twins are on their way, yet later on only one baby is born.

**Vaginal bleeding in the first trimester**
A "threatened" miscarriage, when there is blood loss but the cervix does not dilate and the pregnancy continues, is a sure sign of the interuterine death of a twin. If there an abortion attempt resulting in bleeding and the loss of fetal tissue yet a baby is born, that is a sure sign of a lost twin.

**Ultrasound images**
Pictures of a "vanishing twin" are incontrovertible proof

**Events during pregnancy**
A twin pregnancy can be compromised by trauma such as an accident, an infection, surgical treatment or extreme emotional stress. This can cause total loss of the pregnancy or the death of the weaker twin.

## A breech birth
It is possible that a breech birth is a sign of a lost twin, but this would be insufficient proof in the absence of any other indication. Surviving twins who know of their twin commonly have a diffficult delivery, whether breech or not.

## An unusual placenta
After birth the placenta may be double or of an unusual shape, or very thick. When the placentas of a pair of twins implant close together, they may become fused into one large one, which is retained even after one twin dies.

## Attachments to placenta
Nodules, additional cords or sacs may be found attached to the placenta at birth. They are all that remains of the twin.

## The fetus papyraceous
This is the mummified body of the lost twin delivered along with the placenta. The tiny body is sometimes fused with the placenta, very small and easily missed. Until relatively recently, it has not been usual to mention this to the parents at birth, so it may be more common than it appears. It is now common practice to examine the placenta carefully, so the presence of a fetus papyraceus at birth is now more commonly seen and recorded.

## The fetus in fetu
It can happen very early in an identical twin pregnancy that one twin becomes absorbed into the other and continue to grow inside the body of the other. The twin may not be detected until some health problem is investigated. The twin (sometimes called a *parasitic twin*) is surgically removed.

## A teratoma
If stem cells from a lost twin begin to grow in the body of the survivor then a cyst may develop that has no human form but may contain teeth and hair. Teratomas are referred to as *dermoid cysts* when they are found in the skin.

**Mirrored organs**
Displaced organs in the survivor, particularly the heart on the right side, is a sign of "mirror" twinning- a form of identical twinning with twins who are mirror images of one another. It is possible that left handedness is also a result of this.

**Split organs**
A double uterus, in fact doubling of any organ, such as additional fingers or toes, including additional bones in the spine, are all signs of intrauterine twinning

**Uncertain sexuality**
A person who is genotypically male but with additional female organs or secondary sexual characteristics, or vice versa, may be a surviving twin.

**Genetic chimera**
Where an adult has two different genetic cells lines in their body, they are most probabaly a surviving twin and some stem cells from the lost twin have become lodged in some part of their body and have continued to develop. Some people are blood chimeras.

**Twin- twin transfusion**
Twins who share a blood supply are vulnerable if one twin dies and the blood pools in the dead body of the other, causing acute anaemia in the living twin. This sometimes resolves naturally, leaving a sole survivor with some problems due to a lack of oxygen in the blood.

**Cerebral palsy**
Research seems to show that people with cerebral palsy are surviving twins who suffered brain damage because of twin-twin transfusion early in pregnancy.

# C : SURVIVING TWINS
# AND WOMBTWIN SURVIVORS:

## RESEARCH QUESTIONNAIRE
*(Note: This questionnaire may be photocopied for mailing)*

To help us with our research, this can be completed and returned to
Wombtwin Survivors, PO Box 396, St Albans, Herts AL3 6NE, UK
or faxed to +44 (0)1727 765832
*(can also be completed online on www.wombtwin.com)*

| | Y | N |
|---|---|---|
| **MOTHER'S PREVIOUS PREGNANCIES:** | | |
| No of mother's previous pregnancies resulting in loss of pregnancy or death of the baby (if yes, write no. in box) | | |
| Nature of the loss (miscarriage, abortion, stillbirth, etc.) ............................................................................. | | |
| **INDICATORS DURING YOUR MOTHER'S PREGNANCY OF A POSSIBLE TWIN WITH YOU:** | | |
| Mother abnormally large around the waist in the first three months | | |
| Bleeding in the first three months | | |
| Miscarriage or suspected miscarriage but pregnancy continued | | |
| Attempted abortion but pregnancy continued | | |
| Mother took Clomid or other drug to stimulate ovulation | | |
| Ultrasound evidence of a second gestational sac | | |
| More than one embryo implanted after IVF | | |
| Mother took oestrogen during pregnancy | | |
| A doctor, or nurse suspected a twin pregnancy | | |
| Another person suspected a twin pregnancy | | |
| Other indications ............................................................ | | |

|  | Y | N |
|---|---|---|
| **ASPECTS OF YOUR BIRTH:** | | |
| My birth was traumatic | | |
| Breech birth | | |
| Small for dates | | |
| Placenta unusually large | | |
| other; | | |
| **SIGNS OF YOUR TWIN AFTER BIRTH:** | | |
| My twin was born with me but was stillborn | | |
| My twin was born with me but died in the first 6 months of life | | |
| My twin was born with me but died aged more than 6 months | | |
| Additional sacs or cords were found attached to the placenta after delivery | | |
| Fetus papyraceous present | | |
| Marks or lesions on the placenta | | |
| Other signs of my twin | | |
| **BODILY INDICATORS THAT YOU MAY BE A WOMBTWIN SURVIVOR:** | | |
| Dermoid cyst | | |
| Teratoma | | |
| Fetus in fetu | | |
| Split organs | | |
| Congenital abnormality | | |
| Presence of sex organs or secondary sexual characteristics of opposite sex (details) .................................................................. | | |
| Left-handed | | |
| Ambidextrous | | |
| Cerebral palsy (if YES indicate severity 0-4)          0  1  2  3  4 | | |

|  | Y | N |
|---|---|---|
| Blood chimera | | |
| Other birth defects ......................................................... | | |
| **OTHER FACTORS ASSOCIATED WITH TWINNING:** | | |
| There are fraternal twins among my blood relations | | |
| There are identical twins among my blood relations | | |
| I have always had a great interest in twins | | |
| All my life I have had the feeling that I may have once been a twin | | |
| As a child, I had one or more imaginary playmates | | |
| **IDENTICAL OR FRATERNAL?** | | |
| I know that I am the survivor of an identical (monozygotic) twin pair | | |
| I know that I am the survivor of a fraternal (dizygotic) twin pair | | |
| I am not sure, but I believe my twin was fraternal | | |
| I am not sure, but I believe my twin was identical | | |
| **TRIPLET SURVIVORS:** | | |
| I am one of a twin pair but one triplet died | | |
| I am the sole survivor of a triplet set | | |

## The way you feel about your twin, yourself and your life:

|  | Y | N |
|---|---|---|
| I suffer from depression | | |
| I have always felt as if I had a twin out there somewhere | | |
| I fear abandonment or rejection | | |
| I have considered suicide more than once in my life | | |
| I am afraid of being alone in the dark | | |
| I sometimes feel unable to cope with life | | |

| | Y | N |
|---|---|---|
| I have been searching for something all my life, but I don't know what it is | | |
| I get very intense and involved at the start of a relationship but then I sabotage it somehow | | |
| I am female but I have a strong male side | | |
| I am male but I have a strong female side | | |
| I grieve deeply and for a very long time after someone close to me, or a beloved pet, has died | | |
| Deep down, I feel very vulnerable, as it would not take much to totally annihilate me as an individual | | |
| I am easily bored | | |
| I think a lot about death and dying | | |
| I willingly participate in particular activities that potentially could damage my wealth or well-being | | |
| All my life I have been pretending to be someone else, and I know it's not my authentic self | | |
| I feel the pain of others as if it were my own | | |
| Deep down, I feel alone, even when among friends | | |
| I easily get into a love/hate relationship with individuals I want to get close to | | |
| It upsets me if I am unable to reduce the suffering of others | | |
| I often find it difficult to fall asleep, even when I am very tired | | |
| I am very active, always doing too many things, all at the same time | | |
| There are two very different sides to my character | | |
| All my life I have felt in some way "incomplete" | | |
| I spend a lot of time talking to myself in a mirror | | |
| I find disappointment very painful | | |
| I think I am psychic | | |

# QUESTIONNAIRE

| | Y | N |
|---|---|---|
| I am a perfectionist | | |
| I tend to hold on to things | | |
| I have been in an exploitative relationship with another person | | |
| All my life I have felt an emptiness inside | | |
| I don't let other people get close to me | | |
| I am always feeling paranoid about silly things | | |
| I feel driven by "musts" and "shoulds" | | |
| I get extremely upset over silly little things | | |
| I have a long-term problem with food and eating | | |
| I feel different from other people | | |
| I have a prevailing sense of irrational guilt | | |
| I always feel unsatisfied but I don't know why | | |
| I know I am not realising my true potential | | |
| I have strong, inner imaginary life, that I use as a coping mechanism | | |
| Deep down, I somehow know I experienced death before I was born | | |
| I find it hard to let go of unfinished projects | | |
| I have a strange, irrational feeling that somehow "I don't exist" or "I'm not really here". | | |
| I feel very privileged, simply to be alive | | |
| I generally lack energy and motivation | | |
| There is at least one room (including shed or garage) in my home that is completely full of my stuff. | | |
| I suffer from low self esteem | | |
| I have a problem with expressing anger - either there is too much or too little | | |
| I often feel torn in two between two decisions | | |

|  | Y | N |
|---|---|---|
| I have suffered for a long time from feeling vaguely unwell, as if I am slowly dying | | |
| I make a lot of effort to protect my privacy | | |
| I am so intuitive and empathetic that it is a problem for me | | |
| All my life I have felt restless and unsettled | | |
| All my life I have carried deeply felt emotional pain that persists, despite all my efforts to heal myself | | |
| I feel personally responsible for events that actually have nothing to do with me | | |
| I feel guilty about being alive at all | | |
| I have ambivalent feelings about seeing myself in a photograph or movie | | |
| I want to succeed but I always end up somehow sabotaging my chances of success | | |

Please add any further information on a separate sheet.
Thank you.

~~~~~

The results of this survey will be
discussed in a forthcoming publication:

*"Wombtwin Survivors"*
by Althea Hayton

complete this survey online at
**www.wombtwin.com**

Lightning Source UK Ltd.
Milton Keynes UK
09 December 2010

164086UK00001B/7/A